W9-BTL-450

I'm Here To Help

A GUIDE FOR CAREGIVERS, HOSPICE WORKERS, AND VOLUNTEERS

M. Catherine Ray

BANTAM BOOKS

New York Toronto London
Sydney Auckland

I'M HERE TO HELP
A Bantam Book/April 1997
Previously published by Hospice Handouts
a division of McRay Company in November 1992.

All rights reserved.
Copyright © 1997, 1992 by Hospice Handouts, McRay Company.
Cover design copyright © 1997 by Belina Huey.
Photograph on page 5 by David Deal.

No part of this book may be reproduced or transmitted in any form
or by any means, electronic or mechanical, including photocopying,
recording, or by any information storage and retrieval system,
without permission in writing from the publisher.
For information address: Bantam Books.

Library of Congress Catalog-in-Publication Data

Ray, M. Catherine.
I'm here to help : a guide for caregivers, hospice workers, and
volunteers / M. Catherine Ray.
p.   cm.
Includes bibliographical references.
ISBN 0-553-37797-3
1. Terminal care—Psychological aspects—Handbooks, manuals, etc.
I. Title.
R726.8R38   1997   96-26981   CIP
616'.029—dc20

Published simultaneously in the United States and Canada

*Bantam Books are published by Bantam Books, a division of Random
House, Inc. Its trademarks, consisting of the words "Bantam Books" and
the portrayal of a rooster, is Registered in U.S. Patent and Trademark Office and
in other countries. Marca Registrada. Bantam Books, 1540 Broadway, New York,
New York 10036.*

PRINTED IN THE UNITED STATES OF AMERICA

BVG   10   9   8   7   6   5   4   3   2

HOSPICE PROFESSIONALS PRAISE
I'M HERE TO HELP

"Catherine Ray's book is a treasure! Finally, a book that clearly summarizes vitally important listening and communication skills, not just for hospice workers, but for everyone. The book's format is 'reader-friendly' and could be used in a variety of training settings, including health care institutions, religious communities and businesses."

—Edward Holland
Coordinator of Spiritual Care and Grief Support
Methodist Hospital Hospice, Minneapolis
President, 1993 and 1994,
Minnesota Hospice Organization

"This is the *best* guide I have seen! We will give each new volunteer a copy at our next hospice training."

—Anne L. Walker, Executive Director
Hospice of Marshall County, Guntersville, Ala.

"This clear brief volume, rich in helpful material about self-awareness and family dynamics for hospice workers, supplies many useful examples of initiating and sustaining verbal and listening interactions. It also lists useful references and suggestions for finding and developing reading and related resources."

—Madalon O'Rawe Amenta
Editor, *The Hospice Journal*

Also by M. Catherine Ray

I'M WITH YOU NOW
A Guide Through Incurable Illness for Patients, Families, and Friends

Available wherever Bantam Books are sold

I wish to acknowledge the many people in my
workshops whose experiences and stories contributed to these pages.
Additionally, I'm grateful to the members of my
own hospice program at Methodist, and
especially to the people who have permitted me
to play a part in their personal dying
and bereavement.

PREFACE

Not long ago, a close friend called me from work. She is a personnel supervisor and she described an unusual dilemma.

> "This employee, 'Larry,' has worked here for years and now he's dying of cancer. Friday's his last day, so we're having a party for him. His manager asked what he wanted written on his cake, and Larry told him, 'Enjoy yourself—and with an exclamation mark.' Now I'm supposed to order this cake, and the place is all in an uproar. People say his manager must have misunderstood what Larry said—but they're too embarrassed to ask him again. I personally don't see what's so strange about it, but I finally told them I knew someone who worked with hospices, and I'd get an outside opinion. What do *you* think about all this?"

My friend didn't know if Larry was in hospice. But he certainly embodied the hospice philosophy: he focused on living while respecting his dying as a normal, natural transition. I only hope his managers get the message.

I have faith that they will. The hospice philosophy spreads with each family it touches. Small wonder that the number of hospice programs has more than doubled in my home state of Minnesota since I presented my first hospice workshop in 1985. Hospice makes a difference; nationwide statistics prove it as much as the personal stories one hears.

I'm Here to Help was written for the people who are responsible for that growth—the hospice volunteers and professionals who, on any given day, are helping thousands of families live with dying.

Such people are among the most life-loving humans I know. They are nondefensive and sensitive—a disproportionate percentage of "feeling types" is drawn to this work. Hospice workers are plateaus beyond initial fears and embarrassments; they are comfortable with life's complexities. They share a healthy acceptance of death and dying, and most have superb senses of humor.

They are often asked why they do what they do by skeptical friends and family.

The answer is simple: hospice workers get to eat cake with people like Larry.

Enjoy yourself!

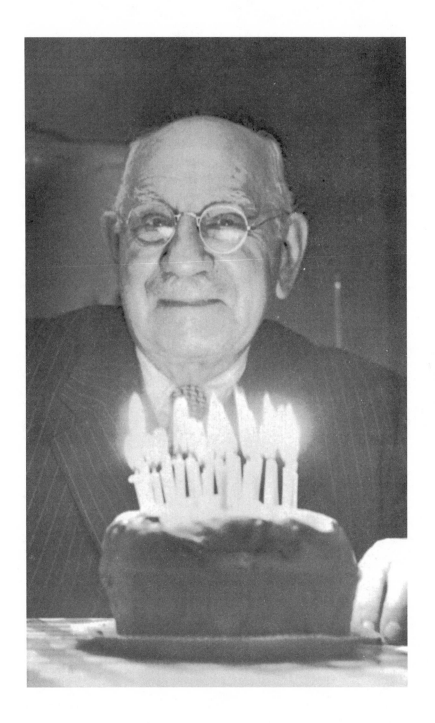

ABOUT THIS BOOK

I'm Here to Help is a book for hospice workers—caregivers, volunteers, and paid professionals alike—anyone on the team who communicates with dying people and their loved ones. The tips and techniques covered have been evolving since my first hospice workshop in 1985. Since then, I've presented many more seminars, become a hospice volunteer, and most important, experienced the loss of loved ones. I decided to compile the information I've collected, to offer a written version of what's in my head and in my workshops.

I didn't see the need to replicate the wonderful books and essays I've read on hospice philosophy, death, dying, and bereavement. Instead, I wanted to provide something I *hadn't* read . . . a handbook of those specific communication skills necessary in hospice, backed by interpersonal communication principles, models, and theory.

Therefore, *I'm Here to Help* is intentionally succinct—as practical and concentrated a presentation as possible, given the complexity of the subject matter. I use a short "pointer" format, intended to be both hands-on and reader friendly. There are few extended examples or explanations.

I hope that new volunteers will read this book during training. I hope that seasoned volunteers and paid professionals will use *I'm Here to Help* for an occasional refresher. In short, I wish to expand the audience beyond those hospice workers I meet in my training classes.

Readers of this book are undoubtedly similar to the people in my workshops—you already intuitively know and practice much of what I'm about to present. You also have ideas to add; in fact, several pointers in this book originated from workshop participants. Hopefully, *I'm Here to Help* consolidates what you already experience, offers new ideas, and also provides an avenue for sharing your own skills and strategies.

CONTENTS

I'm
Here
To
Help

1

PHILOSOPHICAL AND SPIRITUAL APPROACHES

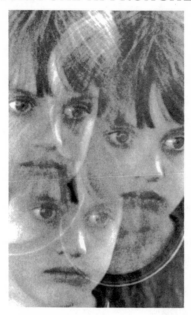

- **Avoid offering definitions of death, the hereafter,** etc. However, encourage the other person to define this experience, spiritually or otherwise, with no argument from you.

- **Try not to deny the reality of somebody else,** for example, by saying to them, "Oh, come on now, you can't really mean that!"

- **Remember that the famous Five Stages of Death are ever changing.**

  Denial ▸ *Anger* ▸ *Bargaining* ▸ *Depression* ▸ *Acceptance*

  No one ever goes through this process entirely predictably or completely chronologically.

- Just as they change **physically**—and sometimes drastically—week to week, patients also change **spiritually** and **philosophically.** You do not see the same person today that you saw four days ago.

- **These philosophical and spiritual changes occur in loved ones, too.**

- **Remember that each friend and family member has a unique relationship** and carries a unique perspective regarding the dying loved one.

- **Do not attempt to share someone's grief,** and be wary of overdoing the empathy. People get very protective and possessive of their grief.

- **Accept human diversity:**

  - **Culture determines what is appropriate interpersonal behavior.** For instance, Native Americans may avoid eye contact as a sign of respect, and an Anglo-American might label those averted eyes unassertive or even deceitful. A reserved European-American might seem closed or controlling to a more expressive, confrontational African-American. Be wary of stereotyping.

  - **Personality preferences play a part.** You might find it energizing to be around others while another person needs solitude to restore the batteries. She might be more logical while he is more emotional. You prefer a set agenda while he operates more spontaneously (See Keirsey and Bates, *Please Understand Me*).

  - **Communication styles will differ.** You might have a *fight* approach while he prefers to take *flight* ("Let's just get the cards on the table" versus "Can't we just sleep on it and try to have a good time tonight?"). He is quite expressive nonverbally and physically demonstrative; she is reserved and prefers to keep her distance. (Note: Often these people are married. Happily.)

- **Become tolerant,** if not comfortable and enthusiastic, about a wide range of rituals/beliefs surrounding life, death, and the dying process.

- In a world plagued by AIDS, hospice caregivers must **examine our own philosophies** regarding sexuality and drug abuse. Do we have religious/spiritual foundations that might pose a barrier?

- **In no way impose your own values, attitudes, and beliefs onto patients and their families.** Are there areas/issues where you might feel judgmental?

- **Broaden your experience by exploring other cultures** and their definitions of death and dying. Read, talk to people of different faiths and nations, and attend their ceremonies.

NOTES

HOSPICE AND
HUMAN DIVERSITY

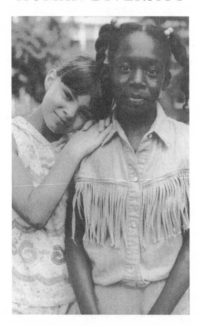

- **At this writing the vast majority of hospice care is provided for white American families by white American hospice workers—predominantly females.** Further, our current hospice practices are decidedly steeped in Christian philosophies about illness, death, and grieving. As we work to increase access to hospice care, it is imperative that we broaden our knowledge and approaches. (The National Hospice Organization has excellent, up-to-date information about our nation's population and access to hospice care—see Resources.)

- **Cultural differences about death and its meaning are vast.** For a Jewish family, it might be inappropriate to send flowers to honor the deceased. For a Hmong family, there may be vitally important family rituals surrounding good spirits and evil spirits entering the body of the deceased and affecting its afterlife. And within a Christian framework, there are major denominational differences.

- **When opening ourselves to new, strange, or foreign ways of living and dying, it helps to remember other differences between us.** Below is a random list of values, concepts, and other elements important to human life. Think carefully of the very different ways various people view them—give yourself at least a few moments to consider every single one. For example, Japanese culture is more collective and group-oriented than that of the "rugged American individualist." Some Native American nations might find the concept of land ownership preposterous, from a spiritual perspective.

   > time   achievement   honor   work   wealth   material gain
   > the afterlife   self-reliance   family   change   success
   > the future   territory   God   leadership   assertiveness
   > nature   sexuality   competition   practicality   trust
   > marriage   individuality   community   formality   friendship
   > informality . . .   and more

- **Training ourselves to understand and even appreciate our diversities is more complex than it might appear.** We are so much more than just our race, or ethnicity, or gender, or religion, or class, or sexual orientation—we are each unique combinations of many attributes. For instance, we run the risk of seriously polarizing ourselves when we think, "I am a white person working with a black family—how should I act?"

- **This type of thinking also casts aside so many other fundamental variables.** In the last example, for instance, it's true that our complexions might be a major difference. But it is *also* important that I am Unitarian while the family is Methodist; I come from a blue-collar family while the patient has few financial concerns; I am heterosexual and the patient is gay; I am a woman and the patient is a man; I am an only child with few relatives and his family has an extensive network of relatives and friends, and so forth. Each of these differences, together with countless others, will affect the ways we understand each other.

- **Many hospice programs choose to handle the topic of cultural diversity in an additive way.** Out of a ten-week volunteer training course, for instance, one week is devoted to "other cultures" and that's the extent of the training. While this is perhaps better than no training at all, it is far from sufficient.

• **The topic of diversity needs to be integrated into every single part of a training curriculum—not merely allocated its three-hour block of time.** Further, we need to address these issues in staff meetings, team meetings, and on every organizational level, every single day of the year. Any time this subject arises, even in casual conversation, stop to address it. Ask specific questions in team meetings about patients, staff, and their diversities.

• **Diversity trainers and participants in their programs need a thorough and substantial understanding of *institutional* "isms."** We must fully recognize the systemic policies, practices, theologies, linguistics, economics, and social behaviors that exclude diverse individuals. For instance, it is a significant institutional policy that American women and black Americans had to fight for the right to vote. Many people in the 1990s weren't personally involved in these historical policies, but the history itself continues to have a profound systemic effect on us all, decades later.

• **When training staff—both paid and volunteer—it helps to expect defensiveness.** Cultural diversity is a potentially volatile topic. It is ambiguous and confusing, and participants often engage in power battles with each other and with the facilitators. People often feel personally attacked—"I'm *not* a racist!"—and misperceptions are common. Whenever we feel defensive, it is harder for us to hear others.

• **Talking about isms (racism, sexism, classism, ageism, etc.) as *institutional* rather than *individual* can help reduce this defensiveness.** If every time we use the noun *racism* we add the adjective *institutional,* people seem to feel much less personally attacked. Saying "White people play a major role in an institutionally racist system" is much less agitating than claiming, "White people are racists."

- **Things will be less stressful if participants want the training; effective facilitators work first to achieve this objective.** Outcomes will not be as positive if staff feel they have to be there, or if they are told they are believed by others to be "prejudiced and insensitive" and thus need the training (even when this is indeed the case).

- **Whenever possible, diversity trainers work with *teams* of facilitators,** representative of a wide variety of cultures. At the same time, it is important to stress that no individual is a final-word spokesperson for every member of the "group" he or she represents.

- **The concept of *assimilation* is an essential ingredient in any diversity training.** We need to acknowledge that a more powerful group often expects those with less power to "get with the program," to learn standard English, to dress in a certain way, to adopt an eight-to-five work ethic, to discipline their children in socially sanctioned ways, to be "on time," and more. For instance, it might be unsettling for an Anglo-American volunteer to work with a Nigerian family and discover that the husband fervently believes his wife became ill because an evil spell was cast on her. This *doesn't* make the husband wrong or "crazy"; he is merely operating from a radically different set of fundamental beliefs.

- **When people don't assimilate, we sometimes exclude them entirely, or at the very least "marginalize" them.** To marginalize someone means to see only a small *part* of the person and to push him or her to the outskirts of our lives. For instance, a close friend of the patient is a Muslim woman who wears a veil. We assume she's in some way subservient or, at the very least, religiously and politically different from us, and we're unsure about striking up a conversation with her because we prejudge her as being on a "completely different wavelength."

- **When we marginalize, we often justify our excluding behavior by calling it *their* fault.** In this "blame the victim" manner we might say, "We *wanted* to help this family with their insurance problems, but they never bothered to learn English well enough . . . the phone calls were just impossible . . . they just couldn't understand our language, much less our health care system."

- **Whenever we find ourselves frustrated by an accent or cringing at unusual grammar, it helps to remind ourselves that the speaker is bilingual** and at least somewhat functional in our language . . . are we functional in *his?*

- **It helps when people with institutional power are able to consider their privileges . . . and acknowledge them.** An excellent and thought-provoking article by Peggy McIntosh highlights this essential idea. The author notes that because she is white, she enjoys certain conditions and advantages that make her life easier . . . and she takes them for granted unless she consciously considers them. McIntosh is adamantly clear that this is merely *her* list, from her experience — these are not the privileges of white people in general. And she encourages every reader to think about and create his or her unique list of privileges. For example:

  - I can arrange to be in the company of people of my race most of the time and avoid spending time with people I was trained to mistrust and who have learned to mistrust my kind, or me.

  - If I should need to move, I can be pretty sure of renting or purchasing a dwelling in an area in which I would want to live and that my neighbors in such a location will be neutral or pleasant to me.

  - I can go into a supermarket and find the food I grew up with, into a hairdresser's shop and find someone who can deal with my hair.

  - Whether I use checks, credit cards, or cash, I can count on my skin color not to work against the appearance of financial reliability.

  - I can be pretty sure that if I ask to talk to "the person in charge" I will be facing a person of my race.

- I can be sure that if I need legal or medical help, my race will not work against me.

- I can be pretty sure that my children will be given curricular materials that testify to the existence of their race.

- I can arrange to protect my children most of the time from people who might not like them.

- I do not have to educate my children to be aware of systemic racism for their own protection.

- I can be pretty sure that my children will be well liked by their teachers if they are obedient.

- I am never asked to speak for all the people of my racial group.

- I can remain oblivious of the language and customs of persons of color, who constitute the world's majority, without feeling any penalty for such oblivion.

- I can turn on the television or open the newspaper and see people of my race widely represented.

- When I am told about our national heritage or about "civilization," I am shown that people of my color made it what it is.

- If I want to, I can probably find a publisher for this piece on white privilege.

- I can do well in a challenging situation without being called a credit to my race.

- I can go home from most meetings of the organizations I belong to feeling somewhat tied in, rather than isolated, out-of-place, outnumbered, unheard, feared, or hated.

- I can be pretty sure that an argument with a colleague of another race is more likely to jeopardize her chances for advancement than to jeopardize mine.

- I can worry about racism without being seen as self-interested or self-seeking.

- I can take a job with an affirmative action employer without having my co-workers on the job suspect that I got it because of my race.

• I can think over many options, social, political, imaginative, or professional, without asking whether a person of my race would be accepted or allowed to do what I want to do.*

• **The label *minority* is a term that bears consideration. The word is deeply imbedded in our national psyche—even in our very laws—but its implications are also potentially divisive and marginalizing.** A colleague once told me, "Why do people in this country *insist* on calling me a minority, when there are far more people in this world who have dark skin like mine than white Europeans? And just think what the word implies—smaller, lesser. I don't appreciate being dumped into some group of 'smaller, lesser' people. Imagine the farmer with an orchard—he has seven apple trees, two plum trees, and one peach tree. Do we say, 'The farmer has an orchard with a thirty percent minority'? No. We say, 'The farmer has mostly apple trees, some plums, and a peach.' I am not a 'minority'—I am a Puerto Rican."

• **As these examples demonstrate, language has incredible power to shape and alter our perceptions.** Until we understand this, we continue to ridicule people who "make a stink" about being called a girl instead of a woman. Or we complain that people are "too sensitive" when they object to the name of a sports team. Or we say things like, "When I grew up, it was 'colored.' Then it was 'black.' Now it's 'African-American.' What's the big deal, anyway, it's just *words*!"

• **We must assume that no single person is the ultimate authority on the words used to describe any group of people.** For instance, I know many women who abhor being called ladies—and I know just as many who relish the term.

Excerpts from: Peggy McIntosh, "White Privilege and Male Privilege," Wellesley College Center for Research on Women, Working Paper No. 189, 1988.

- **Respect the power of language by allowing people to explain why they prefer some words and phrases over others.** And even if you do not agree, accept their perspectives and adapt to their preferences when in their presence. If someone says he doesn't want to be called a "jock," don't argue with him that the word has merit or that "it doesn't really matter" — *just stop using the term.*

- **Accept the labels others assign to their relationships.** Nearly any hospice worker can think of a time when, weeks into visiting the family, she discovered that the patient's "sister" was not a sister after all. Think, too, of the gay man describing his long-term relationship: "Something that really bothers me is when my hospice team refers to Rick as my *friend.* I know they do this because they don't know what else to call him, but the word seems so demeaning when I think of what he is to me. Rick is my lover, my soul mate, my partner, my spouse . . . we've been together twenty-four years and I couldn't be doing this without him. He is so much more than my *friend.*"

- **When trying to figure out what to call somebody, *ask.*** Yes, we feel shy about doing so, but this one-sentence moment of awkwardness saves hours of nagging doubts — and possible offense — throughout the remainder of our interactions. Try saying, "Larry, I can see Rick is a most special person to you. What would be the best way to introduce him to other members of the team?"

- **When in doubt about whether to use formal or informal titles, be safe — opt for a formal approach. Think respect *first*, familiarity later.** This is especially true when there are generational differences between you and a patient or loved one. As one caretaker said, "Everyone is a little uncomfortable when the nurse comes to visit, because she calls Grandma 'Elaine.' You see, no one calls Grandma that. She's either 'Grandma Burr' or 'Mrs. Burr.' She's sort of the matriarch of the community. No one *ever* calls her 'Elaine' except the nurse. So we can't help but notice."

- **To open ourselves to other cultures and ways of thinking, it is most important to think deeply about ourselves.** Rather than look for a checklist of dos and don'ts for a given group of people, we need to look inside to discover what makes us who we are. What values, attitudes, behaviors, and stereotypes do we bring to any interaction? How does our own cultural and spiritual heritage affect our lives?

- **Finally, hospice workers are most helpful when they forge ahead to discover new ideas and ways of living, and they also forgive themselves when they display ignorance or make a cultural gaffe.** It takes years of experience to perceive the intricacies and nuances of cultures, ideas, and spiritual interpretations that are new to us. We must remember to be patient with others, and with ourselves.

NOTES

BOUNDARIES

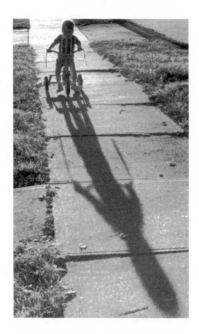

- **Set boundaries.** Observe the suffering and remain compassionate, but don't immerse yourself.

- **Avoid thinking you can solve other peoples' problems.**

- **Be on the lookout for client/family dependency on you.**

- **Learn to say "No."**

- **Be aware of your own "unfinished business"** . . . the things you think and feel about dying, and why. Your own experience with death and dying could negatively affect your work with the family if you aren't careful.

- **Remember that unfinished business goes beyond one's perspective on dying.** For example, imagine that your patient's husband is alcoholic and *you* grew up in an alcoholic family. Take care that your own experience with chemical dependency doesn't negatively affect your work with the family.

- **Avoid becoming the family's therapist.** Are you being pulled in, in ways that feel uncomfortable? Tactfully tell them so.

- **Try not to turn your own family and friends into *your* therapists** (for ways to avoid this, see Chapter 13, "Taking Care of Yourself").

- **I know I'm exceeding my boundaries when:**

  - I lose objectivity . . . for instance, I become resentful toward a family member (even if I don't openly express it)

  - My stress increases . . . I feel emotionally on edge with my own family and friends

  - I find myself thinking about the patient/loved ones too frequently

  - I feel like I want to take over

  - I feel like the patient is *my* responsibility.

NOTES

FAMILY SYSTEMS

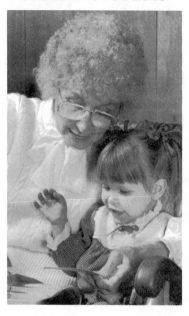

- **The most important people in a person's life are also that person's biggest frustrations.** We are often hardest on those who love us most . . . we trust them not to abandon us, even if we aren't always polite or nice.

- **It is true that opposites attract.** This can be a major source of those frustrations.

- **Continue to learn about family systems and interpersonal communications.** Read books on these subjects, available in the psychology or self-help section of any major bookstore. An even better resource is a textbook on these subjects, available at most college bookstores; these textbooks are quite reader friendly and packed with information.

- **Accept the family wherever they are** in dealing with this experience . . . which will change day to day, from fighting it to accepting it and everything in between.

- Fortunately or unfortunately, **individual family members are rarely at the same collective place** in this process.

- **Each family member brings a unique perspective and plateau** to this experience; each has a unique relationship with the dying person.

- **Watch out for triangle traps.** Do not get hooked between spouses, siblings, parents and children, etc.

- **People have problems above and beyond their illness.** Kids continue to have trouble at school, cars still break down—the little day-to-day irritations of life don't stop when a person has an incurable illness. Instead, they compound the pressure.

- **Families also have major problems . . .** such as financial troubles, chemical dependency, damaged relationships. The functional problems that existed in a family prior to the illness are still there . . . and may even be exacerbated. Do not think these problems can be solved. Deathbed reconciliations do occur, but try to leave romantic illusions at the theater.

- **Families have distinct rules**—even though they probably have not been discussed or formalized—about which feelings/ideas can be expressed. You can tell what things are okay to express by watching various family members as they interact with one another.

- **Families have distinct communication styles.** Just because a family is very loud and argumentative doesn't mean they are unhappy or ready to separate. Just because a family is very reserved and unaffectionate doesn't mean they are uncaring or are "stuffing feelings."

- **Our own family history alters our perceptions of the families we work with.** Again, we must be wary of our own unfinished business.

- **A major comfort the hospice worker provides for a family is the *consistency* he or she offers** to them in a time of great upheaval. Take care to support family routines, rules, roles. Avoid interrupting family patterns (even if you disagree with them).

NOTES

GIVING THE
FAMILY CONTROL

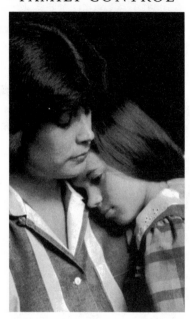

- **When a family joins hospice, they are bombarded with new names and relationships**—social workers, nurses, clergy, home health aides, volunteers. Make it easier for them by wearing a name badge, providing schedule consistency whenever possible, and calling first to confirm visits.

- **Give each and every family member maximum information,** and do not be discouraged or disgruntled when you find your **information has to be repeated or clarified.** People in this situation have difficulty "hearing" because they are already dealing with so much that is new and uncertain. And it is normal that one family member will confuse or distort something you said when repeating it to someone else.

- **Encourage the family in its efforts to educate itself** about the illness and the dying process. Try to be a resource of people, books, and helpful ideas (without soapboxing).

- **Encourage the family to make as many decisions as possible.** For instance, rather than suggesting a menu or scheduling appointments, allow the family to experiment to see which food items work, or how their days are most comfortably organized.

- **When the family is stuck on a problem, first teach them brainstorming** techniques, next help them learn to **prioritize** the most workable ideas, and then **step back** out of the process. Avoid judging the family's perceptions of problems or their solutions.

- **Encourage the family to try something new for a brief time . . .** then help them know that it is okay to change directions. For instance, if the family needs to rearrange living space or alter a diet, suggest, "Let's try this for a few days. If it doesn't work, we'll figure out something new to try."

- **Give family members active and direct permission about losing control** emotionally. Keep tissues handy and don't be shy about handing them out. Affirm emotional reactions directly, saying things like "It's okay to cry. If I were in your shoes, I'd be crying too." At a different time, remind the person how much he or she is accomplishing. (If you compliment people during the time that they are crying, they will think you are merely placating them or trying to make them stop being so emotional.)

- **Learn stress management techniques and when appropriate teach them** to the family so they can better help themselves when team members are not present.

- **People often feel more powerful and in control when they are actively doing something** about a problem. Do not discourage the family from trying to "do things," even if you feel their actions are futile or silly.

NOTES

· 6 ·
HELPING PEOPLE
OPEN UP TO YOU

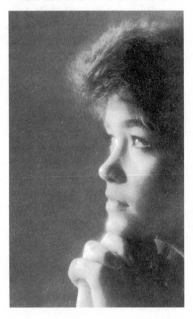

- **Believe what your patient/client and family members tell you . . .** about pain management, coping mechanisms, etc. Do not discount their perceptions or experiences, even mildly.

- Hospice social workers find that major emotional complaints of patients are isolation and boredom. **The hospice worker can become a vital companion.**

- **Do not say "I know how you feel."** This is *not* empathy. It is merely presumptuous.

- **Watch out for the trap, "What would *you* do?"** Often, people will ask for your advice, and not because they really want it, but because it provides them with an opening to talk about their problems. So, instead of answering their question in detail, turn the conversation back to them as quickly as possible. Say something like, "Well, for me, it was like this but I know every family is different. What's going on in *your* situation?"

- **Avoid overdoing descriptions of your own experience . . .** otherwise, you will unintentionally monopolize the airtime.

- **Respect the family's wishes to use euphemisms;** for example, calling incurable lung cancer "my problem." Adjust your language accordingly.

- **Be comfortable as an initiator.** Practice various methods until you can initiate difficult topics with assertive sensitivity.

- **Some initiating techniques are:**

"Can You Tell Me?"	"Can you tell me how your daughter made these cookies?"
The Honest (and Not Overdone) Compliment	"That robe is such a beautiful color—it really brings out the blue in your eyes."
The Whimsical Hook-In	"So, what would *you* name a planet if you discovered it?"
Mutual Interests	"Did you refinish that table yourself? I'm working on a chest of drawers . . ."
External Events	"What did you think of that article in the paper this morning?"
The "Here and Now" Environment	"This room sure gets a lot of sun, doesn't it?"

- If the previous examples seem too commonplace or boring, just remember, **"big talk" usually starts with small talk.**

- **Avoid feeling frustrated or impatient with the same old conversations about the weather, sports, etc.** Such talk (known as phatic communication) provides a vital trust-building function.

- **When initiating difficult topics,** the two rules are:
  1. **Ask permission** to talk about the topic.
  2. **Give the person an "out" at your own expense,** rather than his or hers.

  For example, say "Can I ask a personal question, or am I being a bit too nosy?" rather than "Is it okay to talk about this, or is it just too painful for you?"

- **Use specific and direct initiation questions,** rather than an ambiguous nicety. For example, ask "How did your son react when he found out about your illness?" rather than saying, "If you ever want to talk about anything, just let me know."

- **Do not be too shy to ask scary questions** such as "Are you afraid?" or "What does it feel like to know death is near?" Many patients are grateful for the opportunity to verbalize things that they may withhold from loved ones they want to protect.

- A good way to help the patient talk is to **ask about prized possessions, collections, evidence of hobbies,** etc.

- **Asking to look at photo albums** is another good technique; it can lead to a visit rich with stories, as the patient reviews and celebrates a lifetime of experience and memories.

- If asking to look at photos of family members feels too forward or pushy, try asking to look at **pictures of objects the patient has mentioned:** "Do you have any pictures of that cabin you built?" "Did you ever take any pictures of your garden?" These photos will likely lead to others.

- **Sharing stories is a wonderful tool for gaining trust.** Telling a quick story about yourself will help open the door, but remember that your objective is to hear about *your patients.* Use your stories as a method for evoking theirs.

- **Ask for stories.** "Tell me how you and your husband met." "How did you get started in your career?"

- **Talking is no measure of intimacy.** The closest and most comfortable relationships are ones where we can be together in total silence.

- As the patient approaches death, she sleeps a lot and turns inward, gathering spiritual energy for this important transition. She **expends less energy in here-and-now conversations and interpersonal relationships.** During these quiet times, you can help most by remaining silent, making her comfortable, and holding her hand, stroking her head, etc. (showing her that you are nearby).

- **This sleeping and turning inward can be especially difficult for loved ones.** They may remember an active, vibrant person who was always the life of the party. Family members might complain or worry about the patient's quality of life. Try to help them understand that the patient *is* active, and indeed his life may be taking on a quality more intense than ever. It's just that we can't see it in the ways we did before.

- **The patient may use symbolic language** or speak in ways that seem confusing to caretakers. Often the caretakers may say, "She's rambling."

- This **incoherent, mind-wandering talk is packed with information,** if we listen carefully. The patient may be using metaphors and other symbolic language to communicate two major things: first, what it feels like to die and second, what he needs to make a peaceful exit. (See *Final Gifts,* by Callanan and Kelley.)

- **Listen metaphorically and symbolically**—not just literally (see Chapter 7, "Listening, Feedback, and Managing Conversations").

- **The patient and caretakers do not need to be entertained or distracted** with anecdotes or jokes. Such talk can be trivializing and offensive.

- **It can be really depressing to be with someone who insists on cheering you up.** It takes *so* much effort to be happy for someone, when really we'd rather wallow for a while.

- **Remember that some feelings are more socially acceptable than others.** For instance, feeling anger is more acceptable than feeling fear in our society. Thus, some expressed feelings could be surface ones, masking the real emotions. Someone who seems very angry could be even more scared and sad.

- **Some people view their world more logically, others more emotionally.** (See *Please Understand Me,* by Keirsey and Bates.) In general, it is best to operate within their framework rather than your own. If you are warm/fuzzy/touchy/feely with an analytical person, you'll drive her crazy. If you are all "head" with a "heart" person, he'll view you as cold and aloof.

- **Occasionally, it can be helpful to gently break out of the "head" or "heart" mode.** If someone typically expresses what she thinks, ask also how she feels. When someone expresses feelings, ask also for his thoughts.

- **Sometimes, the very words *thoughts* and *feelings* can be threatening.** If you decide not to be so direct, use a more neutral question: "What was your response to that?" or "How did you react then?"

- **Many patients will confide in a hospice worker things they would never say to a family member or friend.** There is a deep comfort in this short-term relationship, which began with two virtual strangers and no history or preconceived notions.

- At the end of the dying process, many patients have dreams, visions of loved ones who have died, and feelings that they will die soon. Often, patients are afraid to tell their families and friends about these profound experiences because "It will frighten them," "They'll think I'm hallucinating," or "They'll put me in a nursing home." **Hospice workers are often rewarded with hearing these stories.**

- **It is essential for the hospice worker to become a supportive, ethical confidant.** Build trust and acceptance, and know when to keep a secret.

NOTES

7

LISTENING, FEEDBACK, AND MANAGING CONVERSATIONS

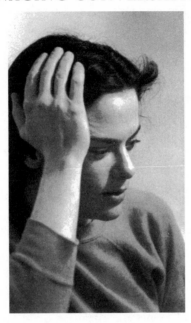

- It's been said before, and for good reason, **Listening is the single most important thing we do.** We must listen well to each family member, and we must listen to each member of the hospice team.

- **Listen with all five senses.** Humans can gather powerful information in every interaction, especially when they pay attention to sight, smell, touch, taste . . . in addition to sound.

- **Listen for literal information, but also listen figuratively.** Patients and caregivers often express themselves through symbols and metaphors; their communication is not always direct or explicit (see Callanan and Kelley, *Final Gifts*).

- **Labels** we give to other people ("bureaucrat," "yuppie," "old maid," etc.) get in the way of our listening to them.

- **Few labels are more emotionally charged than this one: "Dying Person."** By the time you meet them, this label has already altered or eliminated many of the family's former friendships.

• **Loaded language will also get in the way** of open listening. A loaded word is one that carries a powerful emotional punch, such as *chick, imbecile, fag.* Unfortunately, they are different for everybody, so you might use one unintentionally. (Example, "Oh, God!") Take care to choose words that are as value-neutral as possible.

• **Watch out for "naughty" words**—they evoke defensiveness:

You/Your   "**You** didn't call me back to tell me whether I should pick up **your** father's prescription." Instead try: "I was concerned because I wanted to plan for my visit."

Always   **Your** son **always** forgets to call me back." Instead, say: "Many times, I haven't received a call back from Larry."

Never   "She **never** writes out her instructions so I can read them." Instead: "It seems like I have a hard time reading these instructions, too much of the time."

Why   "**Why** do **you** feel that way?" Instead try: "I wonder what brings about those feelings?"

Should   "**You** really **should** talk to a lawyer about revising **your** will." Try instead: "Some people find it helpful to talk to their lawyers about these kind of concerns."

• **The word *you* evokes ego.** Get the ego (you) out of any message which is **correcting**— "I was hoping for a return to my phone call." But keep the ego (you) in when **complimenting**—"You have the prettiest smile!"

• **Avoid changing the subject.** Let the other person do that.

- **Listening occurs at five different levels,** each requiring greater energy and involvement. It's like walking up steps: the higher you climb, the greater your energy and involvement.

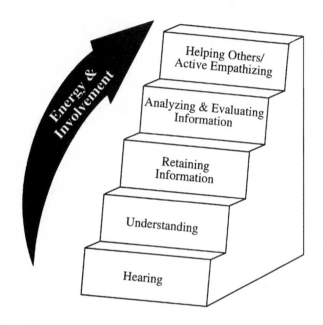

- **Most hospice workers will be required to listen at the top level,** using active empathy and sometimes even counseling skills. This is hard work!

- **Top-level listening is a lot of work,** because you have to hold in your opinions. At this level, you are restricted to using **only nonevaluative feedback techniques** (see Seven Methods for Giving Nonevaluative Feedback, page 35).

- **Nonevaluative feedback means holding back your negative judgments** ("That doesn't sound like it will work!"). It also means **holding back your favorable opinions** ("What a great idea!"). Why hold back our positive feedback, you ask? Because it keeps the person too focused on that one "good" idea and hinders him in exploring other options/thoughts/feelings.

- **Feedback does more than respond . . . it actually changes the messages to follow.** If our feedback judges or evaluates what was said, the speaker will feel compelled to change the message, or perhaps stop talking prematurely. If our feedback is free of evaluation or judgment, we encourage the person to communicate more freely and fully. For example, imagine a conversation with a primary caregiver:

  SHE: I'm just so tired, I think I'll explode.

  YOU: That's such a normal feeling, and nothing to feel guilty about. Perhaps we can arrange some respite care.

  —or—

  YOU: I see. Tell me more about it.

Both responses are good ones, but which one allows the caregiver to solve her own problems (and gives her more control)? Sometimes, counseling communicators mistakenly try to solve other peoples' problems too quickly, before they have had a chance to discuss and solve their problems for themselves.

- **It is important to note that nonevaluative feedback requires more energy and much more time.** In that last example, for instance, it would be harder to say, "Tell me more" if the caregiver made the comment at the end of your visit (and your son was waiting for you to pick him up at soccer practice). Do not feel guilty when you make the decision to refrain from giving nonevaluative feedback.

- **The quickest way to stop a conversation is to provide advice, opinions, evaluations.**

- **Seven Methods for Giving Nonevaluative Feedback**

Minimal Encouragers	Soft murmurs, "Um hm," to acknowledge what is said, while taking little "airtime."
Probing	Ask for more information. "What was your response when he reacted that way?"
Acknowledging	Comment on the behavior of the other in a neutral manner. "I hear some frustration in your voice when you talk about that situation." (Note: You are *not* saying, "I agree. I would be frustrated, too, in that situation.")
Checking Out	Repeat, clarify, reflect, paraphrase. "You say you are confused because this is the fourth time they've changed her prescription?"
Paraphrasing	Use *different* words than the ones the speaker chose, and restate what you heard. This will help both of you to clarify underlying values, hidden attitudes, or unverbalized assumptions. "So, you were feeling angry, or maybe hurt, because he didn't appear concerned?"
Repetition	Use the *same* words the speaker chose, and repeat verbatim what you heard. This will help both of you to clarify specific terms and tangible "contract" issues and to verify the accuracy of statements. "So, her specific words were, 'in ten days to two weeks,' is that right?"
Summarizing	A combination of all the techniques except probing, in which you pull to-

gether the main ideas you heard in a concise paragraph or two. This is a very useful closure technique; it marks the end of your nonevaluative feedback time and helps the person move into evaluating the situation. After your summary statements, you can help the person generate solutions or make decisions.

- **Three Rules for Giving Nonevaluative Feedback:**

  1. **Remember that giving nonevaluative feedback is very tiring.** It is hard to hold back our opinions; this strategy requires tremendous self-discipline and a lot of time.

  2. **Sometimes we evaluate, even when we don't intend to.** Usually this happens through our tone of voice rather than the words we use. To illustrate this, practice all the ways you could say a simple, "Um hmm."

     "Um HMMM . . ." (surprise)
     "Um Hmmmm . . ." (skepticism)
     "UM Hmmm . . ." (agreement)
     "Um Hm . . ." (sarcasm)

  3. **The person receiving nonevaluative feedback will feel validated, and will often believe you agree with what you are hearing.** This can be dangerous! "But you *said* you thought my mother was wrong . . . well, you certainly never *disagreed* with me!"

- **Acceptance is *not* agreement.**

- **Monitor the airtime.** Hopefully, you aren't using much of it.

- **Again, keeping our responses judgment-free requires tremendous attention and self-discipline.**

- **Accept the fact that sometimes you won't have the energy to climb the stairs to top-level listening.** Do not apologize, but do explain: "Marge, I'm distracted right now by outside stuff, but this sounds important . . ." **When you postpone an important conversation, set a *specific* time to hold it at a later date;** "Can we talk about this later?" is not as effective as "Could I come over for coffee tomorrow at seven-thirty?"

- **"Uptones" and "Downtones" are a vocalization technique** that can reduce defensiveness and manage conversational flow. If the last syllable of your sentence goes up in tone, you sound like you are asking a question. If the last syllable goes down in tone, you sound like you are making a statement. For example, say each of these sentences twice, once with an uptone and once with a downtone:

  > "Would you mind if I came on Friday, next week?"

  > "The doctor wants to limit your mother's visitors to immediate fam-i-ly."

  You should be able to hear distinct differences. An uptone sounds tentative, approachable, and inviting. A downtone sounds decisive, powerful, and conclusive.

- **Use uptones when you want to:**

  - encourage someone to keep talking

  - soften the blow of bad news

  - make a statement sound like a question

- **Use downtones when you want to:**

  - conclude a conversation

  - predetermine the response to a specific question

  - make a question sound like a statement

- **Another time management technique is choosing close-ended or open-ended questions.** A close-ended question elicits yes or no, or other short answers, and does not foster further communication.

Close-ended: "What time is your appointment?"

"Ten-thirty."

An open-ended question has no predetermined response and allows the respondent to elaborate.

Open-ended: "What happened when the nurse came by?"

or

"What happened when your daughter told the grandkids?"

- **Use open-ended questions when you want to:**
  - encourage the client/loved one to talk
  - get more information and insight from the client/loved one
  - help the family explore values, problems, possible solutions.

- **Use close-ended questions when:**
  - you want to obtain concise, specific information from the client
  - you want to get the client back on track, conversationally
  - you want to begin the ritual of ending the visit/conversation
  - you sense yourself and/or the client beginning to tire.

- **Hospice workers avoid giving advice,** refrain from judging reactions or decisions, and let patients and loved ones work through the process of dying for themselves.

- **Hospice workers learn to become comfortable with awkward pauses and long periods of quiet . . .** this is especially true toward the end, when the patient turns inward and rests a lot, in preparation for the final departure.

- **Strive to understand,** rather than to be understood.

- **Your biggest gift is frequently your silence.**

NOTES

8

NONVERBAL
TECHNIQUES

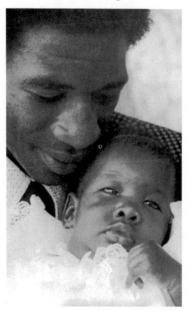

- Pay careful attention to the **environment**—"special" furniture, traffic patterns, privacy issues, etc. Place this family in the context of their surroundings . . . you can gain a lot of information by observing (and respecting) how they use their belongings/surroundings to define themselves. Are doors open/closed? Is there a cluttered/austere appearance? Are conversation areas public/intimate? Respect the family's choices.

- **How we use and define time** is a nonverbal element—the glance at the watch during a conversation, the meeting held at seven-thirty versus the one at noon.—These things are not vocal, but they do shape the interaction.

- **Time is power.** In any relationship, the person who controls the clock has more power. In a job interview, the potential employer can be late; not so the applicant. It is the parent, not the child, who determines how family time is spent (bedtimes, vacation days, doctors' appointments, etc.). It is the boss who determines the time for the meeting, not the employee.

- **Dying people and their loved ones have lost control of the clock.** One moment, they lived with the idea that their futures were more or less infinite . . . the next moment, they came home from the doctor with parameters. This can make people feel powerless.

- **Persons who are not primary caregivers may unintentionally abuse the family's time.** Such people often want to spend time with the patient for their own purposes; they may not realize that the dying person has little energy for interpersonal relationships, especially as death approaches. Hospice workers can help educate the family to set limits, and they can spread the word that a ten-minute visit might be ample.

- We help the family when we **allow them to decide how they spend their time**—being flexible to changing plans, not taking it personally when people prefer not to interact with us.

- **Touch the client often and appropriately . . .** with permission. People with incurable illnesses are not touched as frequently as they were before; we are nervous about hurting them, or worse, disease can carry a stigma. Brush the client's hair, massage his hands, hug her, stroke his arm.

- **Touch is cultural;** some cultures are huggers while some prefer to keep their distance. Be sensitive: avoid overwhelming the family with your affections.

- **Be aware of the potential power trip in touching someone.** In any relationship, the person with more power touches the other person more often. Teachers pat their students' shoulders with familiarity—the student would never be so disrespectful as to return this gesture. Managers congratulate employees with a hearty pat on the back—but employees who did this to the boss would be considered forward. Hospice workers can overdo a good thing if their touching becomes intrusive.

- **Eye contact can also be too much of a good thing.** First, eye contact is culturally determined; some cultures view it as a sign of disrespect. Second, just about everybody needs some private time when face-to-face in conversation. Look away occasionally as the person gathers his thoughts or deals with a complex emotion.

- **Height is power.** Get your head lower than the client's. Use a short stool, sit on the floor beside the couch, lean forward in your chair. Position your face so that you are looking up at the client, rather than down on her. Nurses, though much of their work is performed above the client, can still find sixty seconds or so to crouch by the bed for some gentle conversation.

- **Your chin is the most powerful part of your body.** When your chin is in the air, you are looking down your nose at someone. You appear superior, condescending, or confrontational. (Try it in the mirror and see.) To give the family more power, ever so slightly drop your chin to your chest in each interaction.

- **People who take up a lot of space are more powerful**—big gestures, wide movements, arms akimbo or on hips. You'll empower the family if you tone down your gestures and keep your arms closer to your sides.

- **A pen is a power symbol,** a reflection back to those days when our parents shook their fingers at us. Any sort of pointer or extension held in the hands (such as glasses) operates as a symbol of authority. Hold the pen when you go for a bank loan—put it in your pocket when talking to patients and loved ones.

- **The voice determines power.** Your tone, rate, volume, vocal variety, diction—all can intimidate or invite. A tentative, softer tone can be more calming than strong tones with a lot of vocal variety. However, if you sound sickeningly sweet to a patient/ loved one with a confrontational style, you'll drive him crazy.

- **Mirror the other person.** Match her voice, posture, gestures. Adapt to *her* nonverbal style and preferences to create extra empathy and trust.

- **Learn how to read deceit . . .** and yes, the eyes *do* lie. We are very adept at masking our eyes and facial expressions to pretend that everything is just fine. We are not so adept at remembering to control other parts of our body. We might jiggle our feet or curl our toes, we might pull on our nose or cover our mouth when telling a falsehood.

- **If a person's vocal message contradicts her nonverbal behavior, we believe the nonverbal portion.** For example, the caretaker looks down and sighs as she tells you that her career isn't suffering.

- **How we touch ourselves is a good clue to our real inner state.** Such self-touches are "out of awareness" . . . we don't really realize that we are doing it, and therefore observing these touches can be very helpful for finding the person behind the mask. There are three main types:

  Soothing Self-Touch: Where I stroke my arm or hands, hug myself, or touch myself in other comforting ways when I talk.

  Used when I want to calm myself, tell myself that things will be all right.

  Stimulating Self-Touch: Where I touch myself in more erotic but not taboo places, stroking my own neck, thigh, or lips as I speak.

  Used when I feel alert, happy, involved in the conversation.

  Punishing Self-Touch: If I exaggerated this self-touch, I would inflict pain. I pinch my own arm or bite my thumb, slap my hands together or chew my lip.

Used when I am feeling guilty or remorseful about something. Often in use when I am hiding the truth.

- **Read these self-touches and adapt to them.** Back off or perhaps gently probe—you be the judge—when you see soothing or punishing behaviors. Avoid changing things when you see stimulating self-touches; they are an indication that you are on the right conversational track.

- **Do recognize that these self-touches might not be relevant to the actual conversation you are having.** A neck-pinching primary caregiver may be flashing back on an earlier argument she had with her boss, even though you see the gesture when you are talking about her father. Try not to jump to conclusions.

- **Jumping to conclusions is dangerous** in any event. While nonverbal behavior does account for 65 to 95 percent of the entire message, it is also highly subjective, culturally determined . . . and easy to misread. When assessing a person's motivations or unspoken thoughts/feelings, look for corroborating evidence. Use more than one nonverbal cue and listen to vocal messages when drawing conclusions.

NOTES

9

MANAGING DEFENSIVENESS
AND CONFLICT

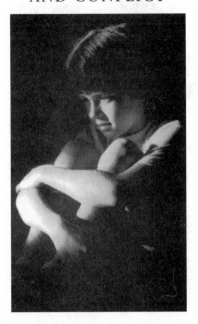

- Remind yourself, and remind your clients, that **venting and anger are normal.**

- **Managing conflict takes energy.** One has to control emotions, listen well, and weigh words carefully. The higher you climb toward resolution, the greater your effort.

- Managing conflict is complicated by the fact that different family members are at **different levels of resolution.** For example, a dying man wants to discuss his estate with a daughter who denies that her father is seriously ill.

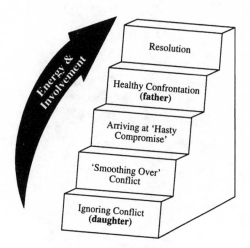

- **There is a cost-reward ratio** in choosing any communication behavior, but particularly in managing conflict. In other words, the rewards have to outweigh the costs, or the confrontation (*behavior*) won't occur.

$$\text{Behavior} = \frac{\text{Reward}}{\text{Cost}}$$

- **Some conflicts are just not worth arguing about.** With others, it seems essential to lay our cards on the table.

- **It would be easier if everyone agreed on the relative rewards and costs of having a given argument!** For example, in that father-daughter situation, the two people have very different orientations toward the same behavior (discussing the estate).

For the **father:**

$$\text{Discussing estate} = \frac{\text{Closure, comfort in planning/decisions}}{\text{Energy needed to deal with daughter's resistance}}$$

For the **daughter:**

$$\text{Discussing estate} = \frac{\text{Pleasing father}}{\text{Facing her own complex emotions, fear}}$$

The father might be so anxious for planning/closure comfort that he is willing to wade through his daughter's resistance. But the daughter's desire to please her father might not outweigh her fears and complex emotions. Thus, the father pushes her to talk about the estate, but the daughter refuses to comply.

• Before we can have a healthy confrontation, **we first have to agree that engaging in the discussion will be worth it.**

• **Fifty percent of all people adopt a flight style when dealing with conflict. Fifty percent of all people adopt a fight style.**

Flight   Easy-going people who do not wish to hurt others, sometimes failing to be totally honest

versus

Fight   Forthright people who express emotion freely, sometimes without tact or discretion

• People in primary relationships (husband and wife, mother and son) often have different preferences—theirs is a **complementary fight-flight relationship.** There are periods of calm and storm—they fight about whether or not they should fight.

• Sometimes, **two fighters** are in a primary relationship. Theirs is a loud, confrontational method of conflict management. They are energized by argument and they fight about everything.

- Sometimes **both parties are flight-takers.** Their relationship appears calm but under the surface, unspoken conflict still exists. They silently wonder if they should fight.

- Fighters accuse flight-takers of "stuffing feelings." Flight-takers accuse fighters of making "mountains out of molehills." **Neither method is better**—they are just different.

- Any time a person has a conflict, he has **only a 50 percent chance of dealing with another person who shares his preference for** fight or flight.

- **People in conflict will inevitably behave defensively.**

- **There is no need to apologize for feeling defensive.** Any time we are scared or anxious, we defend and protect ourselves. Defensiveness is normal, and sometimes even helpful.

- **Would you take away the crutches from a person with a broken leg?** Similarly, don't try to "get rid" of a person's defensiveness. We need our defense mechanisms, at least at the moment of anxiety/fear/anger. Instead, be patient. The leg will heal (with a little help) and the crutches won't always be necessary.

- **Rather than denying a person's right to be defensive, learn to recognize specific defense mechanisms.** This will help you to avoid intensifying them:

    THE RATIONALIZER: Finding reasons to justify an unhappy turn of events.

    "It's actually okay that my father is dying . . . he's old enough to have had a full and happy life."

    Response: Do not discount the explanations/logic of the person, regardless how "crazy" or preposterous. "It's okay that your father is dying?! Oh, come on now!" This will only make the person "explain" even more. Instead, just listen, nod . . . and be sure not to smile (which she would certainly find patronizing).

THE OSTRICH: Totally suppressing any feelings of defeat/conflict. Danger lies in the fact that repressed feelings explode, eventually.

"Tina always seemed to be so cheerful and bright, until I found her sobbing hysterically in front of the TV last night. The sound wasn't even turned on. I was really scared . . . she was the one who was keeping *me* in control."

Response: Do not try to force the person to talk about it. "Tina, you're in denial—it's so obvious. You'll feel so much better if you just talk about this." No, she won't . . . and if you confront her this directly, she'll squirm and probably wish she could run from the room. If you feel you must get her to open up, try to ask very neutral, nonthreatening questions. "So, what kind of a day have you had today?"

THE FINGER-POINTER: Blaming someone else to explain our own fears/failures.

"How can I be expected to put together a decent meal for everyone when I have to spend half the afternoon chasing after *your* father's prescription?"

Response: Do *not* try to get the person to accept blame. "Come on now, no one is looking for a gourmet meal and besides, the pharmacy is only ten minutes away." This will only make the person deny responsibility even more vehemently. Instead say, "It isn't really important how this happened . . . let's just solve the problem. How about if we order a pizza?"

THE COMPENSATOR: "Treating" yourself when things are difficult, threatening, etc.—a basis for serious problems like obesity and chemical dependency.

"The only way I can get through my evening visit to the hospital is to pop over to the mall afterwards. I've bought three pairs of shoes this month."

Response: Do not call attention to the treats. This will not eliminate them; it will only cause the person to hide them. (Obviously, in severe cases such as bingeing, bankruptcy, or alcoholism, intervention is sometimes necessary.)

THE PROTESTER: Publicly taking a position that is the opposite of what you privately feel, because you think your private thoughts are wrong or taboo.

"Why should anyone be afraid of dying? We've *always* believed that God has a better future in store for us!"

Response: Like the Rationalizer, this person will only become more defensive if you point out inconsistencies and illogical statements. Avoid arguing and don't focus on what was said; let the statements slide.

THE REACTOR: Taking out anger or frustrations on something unrelated to the conflict—hopefully an inanimate object, but not always.

"Boy, Rita was really slamming the dishes around last night!"

Response: Do *not* tell the person to calm down. This will only infuriate her even more. Instead, get out of the way! Later, calmly acknowledge apologies and try not to make the person feel any more guilty about damage that was done. Allow her some private time to clean up, repair, and replace. (Obviously, in severe cases of physical/verbal abuse, intervention is in order.)

THE PASSIVE-AGGRESSOR: Acting as if nothing is wrong, but secretly planning on revenge, often to be carried out later.

"Paul has been so charming, even funny lately. Then last night he told me he wouldn't be coming by once a week anymore. I wanted to talk to him about it, but he kept denying anything was wrong."

Response: This is one of the more slippery mechanisms because often the aggression won't occur until days, weeks, or even months after the triggering event, so it is hard to see a connection. It's best to try to find the connection yourself . . . then directly address the aggression and mention a possible triggering event. "It seems like our relationship has changed. Does this have anything to do with that remark I made about your sister?" Unfortunately, you won't always receive a truthful answer, so you might remain confused. But sometimes just acknowledging the aggression or triggering event is enough to make the behavior stop.

- **Do not immediately argue with a defensive person.** Contradicting him will make him even more defensive. Instead, use nonevaluative feedback techniques (see pages 33–38).

- **The best way to manage defensiveness is to expect it, acknowledge it, and avoid intensifying it.**

NOTES

10

TEAM MANAGEMENT

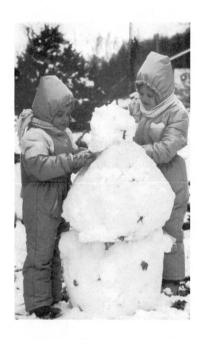

- **Hospice is unlike many other industries in that it operates on principles of collaboration rather than competition.** We try to pool resources throughout our communities, rather than duplicating services. We draw together specialized experts and work in teams, each member bringing a unique perspective to the families we serve.

- **This approach is the beauty of hospice. It is also the cause of major frustrations,** because these very different people have meetings at which they must effectively share information, determine common goals, mutually decide things, and sometimes defer to the judgments of others. These meetings aren't exactly easy.

- **The team meeting is an event found behind the scenes of nearly every hospice.** In these meetings, scheduled on a regular and frequent basis, the nurses, social workers, clergy, volunteer coordinators, patient care coordinators, and others meet to discuss the specific situations of the patients and families they serve.

- **Every team has a personality above and beyond the personalities of its various members.** In other words, the sum is more than its parts. That's why we can like all our co-workers individually, but hate it when they're all in the same room together.

- **It helps to think about the attributes of our own work group.** Are there behaviors and dynamics we'd like to change? Do we enjoy interacting and accomplishing things with our team members? Do we feel good being members?

- **Every group has rules and roles. Sometimes these group *norms* are formalized, sometimes they are not.** For instance, the social worker has a specific job description and so does the nurse—how each member contributes to the team meeting is formally understood, and may even be documented in a job description. But other rules are less explicit—such things as appropriate dress, appropriate use of slang or profanity in a given setting, who speaks first, who speaks longest, the degree of familiarity between members, whether or not these work colleagues socialize. These are informal norms; members just somehow know they must follow them.

- **Most groups have deviants. Deviants are people who don't abide by a rule or role—and sometimes *more than one* rule or role. The greater the number of violations of the norms, the greater the deviancy. . .** and the more frustrating the deviant is to other members. For instance, your team *could* tolerate Barb's perpetual lateness to meetings—if she didn't also insist on mooching everyone's lunch and monopolizing the conversation as well.

- **Sometimes, we don't follow a rule because we don't realize it exists until after we've broken it.** For example, a nurse asks the new social worker if she'd care to contribute to the birthday kitty for another team member. The social worker says, "Not this year.

I don't feel I know her that well yet, and anyway, I like to keep my work and social life separate." At the next team meeting she discovers the group ritualistically holds a small birthday celebration for every team member—and she is embarrassed to find she's the only one who hasn't contributed.

• **Sometimes a deviant breaks a rule or role in open defiance.** She may think the rule is silly, or wrong, or destructive, so she *intentionally* refuses to follow it. This behavior can have several repercussions, both positive and negative.

• **On the helpful side, the deviant might actually turn out to be a change agent . . . the entire organization changes for the better** because she was brave enough to stand up for something significant and make others see its value. For example, the average home-care worker owes a big thanks to Mrs. Amelia Bloomer, the deviant who first wore pants in public—in New York City in 1849.

• **But just as often, deviant behavior can splinter the team.** First, it taxes the group's valuable time and energy. Just to *deal* with the deviancy takes its toll. Team members can grow resentful, and quite quickly.

• **When a team member operates in a deviant manner, other members typically go through an indirect process of trying to eliminate the behavior:**

    • First, the group tries to ignore the deviant's behavior; they attempt to rationalize away its significance. "It doesn't really bother us; it doesn't matter."

    • Second, the group tries to handle the behavior with humor—when it occurs, they make little jokes and chiding remarks, hoping the problem group member will get the hint: "Glad you could finally make it!"

    • Third, open ridicule and sarcasm take over where gentle attempts at humor failed. The group begins to scapegoat and bad-mouth the deviant. "How would you know? You weren't even *here* when we decided this!"

- Finally, the group ostracizes the deviant. They don't include her in the social chit-chat that warms up the meeting; they sometimes "forget" to tell her about important information, upcoming events, and other get-togethers.

- **It might be better if we'd have the courage to add a step between the first and second—call it the direct approach. In a kind but to-the-point manner, inform the deviant about the "rule."** For example, try saying to an overly intimate and talkative team member, "We don't want you to feel hurt and we do think your new house sounds exciting. But we want you to notice that the rest of us don't talk about anything except the patients during team meetings. We just don't have time to talk about our outside lives, right then."

- **By the same token, cohesive groups have a healthy balance of "task" and "social" orientation.** Members feel comfortable about sharing their *whole* selves—not just their work selves. But the socializing has its proper place and boundaries—happy team members come away from meetings with a tremendous sense of progress and accomplishment. They feel their time together is valuable, not frittered away or wasted.

- **Who leads the group isn't always as straightforward as it appears.** And don't let the label *team leader* fool you. Many times a person has a leadership title, but members don't respect that person or treat her as the leader. For example, think of the bosses you've had. Aren't there one or two you found completely incompetent? You officially answered to this boss perhaps, but you chose to go elsewhere for mentoring and guidance.

- **Leadership is earned, not assigned.** Every good leader understands this—she works hard to achieve her responsibilities and to continuously maintain the group's trust.

- **There is no single best style of leadership, just as there is no single best personality style.** There are times to be approachable and times to remain aloof. There are good reasons for democracy, autocracy, even dictatorship. The effective leader develops her own style and assets with practice—and frequently asks group members for their comments on her methods. If it becomes clear that her leadership style damages morale, she makes changes.

- **All leaders have their perfections, all have their flaws.** The good leader merely has more of the former, fewer of the latter. All leaders need help—they need members to contribute to the overall team purpose and also to provide corrective feedback about the group dynamics, aside from the overall purpose. For example, perhaps your hospice is more than effective in managing a census of seventy-five. Aside from that, do you like going to your team meetings? Do you feel nurtured by your co-workers? Do you feel people listen to your opinions? Do you feel the meetings accomplish their objectives, in the most efficient way possible?

- **Many people mistakenly assume that a happy team is one that has no conflicts. This is not true!** A group with no conflicts is impossible. If group members are always outwardly happy and satisfied, they are hiding from each other—they do not trust each other enough to bring up difficult issues.

- **A truly cohesive group is one that has experience with conflict. The team has weathered some internal storms—and they're still together.** They know they won't abandon each other—or their overall purpose—over a disagreement. They trust each other. (Obviously, for conflict to be helpful it must be *healthy*, devoid of nasty tactics—see Chapter 9, "Managing Defensiveness and Conflict.")

- **An agenda for team meetings is a helpful stress-reduction tool; it provides predictability and a sense of accomplishment.** Over time, the schedule of events becomes integrated into members psyches and meetings move smoothly—almost under their own momentum. Some agenda tools that may help are:

- **Have participants determine the format of the agenda, as well as its items and priorities.** Don't allow the leader to impose an agenda on the group or determine the topics for discussion.

- **Use the same format each time.** This provides stability and comfort and helps people indirectly prepare for the meeting in the days between; when something pertinent happens, members consider where in the meeting agenda this issue fits and they mentally rehearse the telling of it.

- **Share the "emcee" duties.** If your format is stable, it is relatively easy to turn over the chairperson responsibilities to different members each time. This technique is empowering, it helps all members appreciate the "big picture," it's fun, and it is a great tool for building responsibility and cohesion.

- **Be open to spontaneous agenda changes.** Provide flexibility for last-minute additions and deletions, be willing to spend more time discussing an issue than originally allocated, and be open to new format ideas.

- **Begin and end on time.** *Always.* Even if the "most important" people aren't there yet, even if an item must be tabled, unfinished, until a later meeting.

- **Continue the meeting** even when someone "important" is pulled away.

- **Begin meetings with a five-minute "cohesiveness" ritual . . .** such as sharing joys and concerns outside of work, talking about the funniest thing that happened that week, or asking a provocative question. Have members *themselves* come up with these rituals. Be sure to limit this time to five minutes, however! Bond, mark the occasion, then move to the task.

- **Encourage creativity.** Make the meetings fun and playful, while simultaneously *productive.* Use lots of structured exercises, such as brainstorming, mindmapping, free writing, and more. (Read books by Roger von Oech, such as *A Kick in the Seat of the Pants* and *A Whack on the Side of the Head.*)

- **Work—like talk—expands to fill the allotted time.** If you give yourselves fifteen minutes to solve a five-minute problem, the task will take fifteen minutes.

- **Save the most difficult topics for last.** Specifically set aside the last fifteen minutes to highlight these—otherwise they will eat up the entire team meeting. When the allocated time arrives, be sure to drop the other topic you are discussing even if it is unfinished. If you don't, members will feel the group isn't willing to deal with difficult issues.

- **Expect unfinished business.**

- **Effective team members are aware that *all* members compromise**—though when there is an especially vocal teammate, it can *appear* she "railroads" decisions and always gets her own way. Any group creates a unique product—an idea, decision, concensus—which is almost always a blending of the contributions of all members but never precisely like that product of any specific individual. Nobody gets his or her own way, at least not entirely. We all compromise, even when it doesn't appear so.

- **We are most motivated to do well when we feel invested in the decisions that affect us.** For instance, we're more willing to abide by punctuality policies if we helped write them. Patient care scheduling is best done by those it most deeply affects—the nurses. We get more from our in-service training when *we* choose the topics—and even sometimes teach the classes. **The effective team gives every member *maximum control.***

- **Effective teams** are stable but fluid, work-focused while playful, easy-going though opinionated . . . and **effective members** are treasured for their maverick originality, tempered by their willingness to blend in when necessary.

NOTES

11

THE HOSPICE
VOLUNTEER

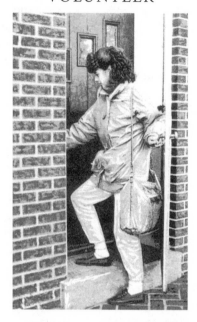

- **The hospice volunteers reading this book—those seasoned and those fresh from training—are in good company.** In 1992, a National Hospice Organization census counted 96,000 hospice volunteers in the United States alone. We gave 5.25 million hours that year. The numbers are perhaps higher today, because hospice in our nation has grown 15 percent in the past two years alone.

- **Hospice couldn't exist without its grassroots volunteer base.** Volunteers started many of the hospices in this country, in fact. Perhaps ten years ago, a retired nurse pooled her skills with a caring committee from her parish and the idea grew from there.

- **Today, hospice volunteers are found through churches, newspaper advertisements, postbereavement social groups, colleges, and more.** It is exciting to think that many hospice professionals are educating our children in elementary and high school . . . and even recruiting them as volunteers. An elementary school child can mow a lawn once a week, or take the patient's dog for a long, daily walk. A college student can be trusted with most routine tasks of patient care, offering the family real respite. Just imagine the internship possibilities that could be sponsored by your hospice—or the Scouts, the school system, the local Y, community colleges, newspapers, libraries, and many other organizations.

- **When recruiting volunteers, two excellent areas to search are local religious organizations and postbereavement groups. However, volunteers with church or grief experience can also overstep their boundaries.** Church volunteers might unwittingly impose their own faith's values on the families they serve—a huge mistake. It is essential to offer more than enough training about hospice and its nondenominational approach to all volunteers, and especially to those recruited from religious organizations.

- **Most hospices prefer volunteers who have experienced the loss of loved ones. But they wisely *won't* accept volunteers with *recent* grief experience.** People in active grief sometimes subconsciously want to work with other grieving people for their *own* purposes . . . to vicariously relive the experience, to process their *own* unresolved issues with grief. And remember, complicated grief can last for *years.* Just because a person's loss came over a decade ago doesn't guarantee she's able to serve a family with the necessary objectivity, even today.

- **Hospice programs sometimes speak of their volunteers as being separate from the other, "professional" members of the team.** For example, a hospice director might say, "We'd like to invite all staff—both professional and volunteer—to this next in-service." The exclusive nature of this language, though unintentional, undermines the contributions of the highly trained hospice volunteer. After all, we are all professionals who serve this family—it's just that some of us are paid and some are not. I personally prefer the phrase, "Paid staff and volunteer staff."

- Of course, hospice volunteers are trained for months—not years, like social workers, nurses, and clergy. It is essential that volunteers everywhere remember that **we are *not* there because of the expertise we can provide to the family.**

- **Instead, volunteers can think of themselves as next-door neighbors—a perspective that keeps us from getting in over our heads.** A neighbor might pick up a prescription, stay with your ill father-in-law, perhaps even help with a bath. But a next-door neighbor doesn't prescribe medicines or answer your Medicare questions; instead, she provides referrals for others who can provide expert help with these matters.

- **A hospice volunteer works within important constraints and boundaries—legal, ethical, and otherwise.** First, she needs to support her hospice program's case management decisions without always fully understanding them—she *doesn't* have access to the patient's medical chart, nor an in-depth perspective regarding state and federal regulatory issues. Second, the good volunteer needs to be supportive and available to the family without getting caught up in their family system. In short, she needs to be approachable, yet able to stand out of the way. It is extremely helpful if she's skilled at minding her own business.

- **A newer hospice volunteer will undoubtedly encounter moments when she feels ill-equipped to do the job.** For example, she needs to move the patient—a *heavy* patient—and she feels awkward as she racks her brain trying to remember what she learned the night "transfers" were covered in her training classes. This first-time fear is a completely normal reaction, and any volunteer out in the field should be comforted to know that she can call her program for help and advice, twenty-four hours a day.

- **This lack of expertise is also a major advantage, as a volunteer may discover within the first few weeks of this work.** The typical hospice volunteer empowers the family far more than the program's paid staff members—because the volunteer is the only person on the team who knows even less than the family members do. This strange paradox helps families bond with their volunteers in a way they can't with those "expert" nurses and social workers on the team. It is much easier for a volunteer to turn over control to the family.

- **Time after time, in my work as a hospice volunteer, I see patients and their loved ones literally turn into different people when a paid professional (such as a nurse, social worker, or volunteer coordinator) walks in the door.** Suddenly the family's voices become childlike, body postures become submissive; there are more uptones at the ends of sentences as family members ask questions and seek reassurance. Watching this transformation, I think to myself, "Just thirty minutes ago, these people were talking to *me* with power and authority. The paid professional arrived, and the family turned into jelly!" When the nurse leaves, family members change back again, into people who are self-confidently educating *me* about their illness and symptom management. The change is remarkable.

- **It's as if this family has two distinct personalities—and, in fact, it *does!*** When the nurse is there, family members are students. When the nurse leaves, family members are teachers. The nurse sees more anxiety, a volunteer sees more clarity and confidence. Nurses and social workers need to remember that patient families are often *much* stronger and *much* more powerful than they appear.

- **Another major advantage of the volunteer role is the lack of an agenda.** When a nurse comes to call for a routine visit, she might be able to allocate an hour—if it's a less busy day. Her time with the family is *focused*—each week, they discuss pain medications, nutrition, elimination, mobility. The volunteer, on the other hand, arrives at the door—perhaps to stay for a luxurious three or four hours—and says, "What shall we do today?"

- **This gift of time, with no set agenda, means the volunteer's relationship with the family can freely meander all over the**

place. Hospice volunteers hear more stories, look at more photographs. They often see a much richer picture of the family than anyone else on the team. And because they typically work with just one family at a time—not twelve or fifteen, like the typical hospice nurse—they have time to notice the nuances. That's why hospice volunteers are the eyes and the ears of the team.

- **The effective volunteer documents her visits, and promptly.** Volunteers must appreciate that any certified hospice program complies with a host of policies—insurance, medical, ethical, and otherwise—and any person who has contact with a patient family is expected to account for his or her actions. Many hospice programs have developed a checklist visit report form with a self-addressed/stamped envelope to make this task easier on volunteers.

- **A helpful volunteer writes up her visits with concise clarity, and also remembers that her words become a part of the family's permanent file.** As such, they could be publicly scrutinized by other agencies in the future. It is important to remain descriptive rather than judgmental and to think carefully about including extremely sensitive or confidential material. Perhaps it is wiser to turn to your Volunteer Coordinator and convey such information verbally, and then discuss if it ought to be included in the written file.

- **Every hospice volunteer knows that what she does with her spare time can be a social conversation-stopper.** People look incredulous, sad, pitying, admiring—all these reactions flit across their faces simultaneously. It can be confusing; we don't know which one to pick or how to respond. Invariably, their next remark will be, "I could never do that—how can you do that? It takes a very special person to do what you do." After a while, a hospice volunteer hears those words more times than she can count.

- **I don't think the adjective is even *accurate*. We aren't such "special" people—the word *special* just removes us from others.** It places us on a pedestal and gives other people a ready excuse to say they couldn't do this type of work, even before they allow themselves to consider trying.

- I'm a hospice volunteer myself—and one with a profound sense of the job's "calling"—so I hope it's clear I'm *not* demeaning us when I say **anybody can do what we do.** Yes, maybe we're a little more patient—because we've spent twenty minutes helping someone walk ten feet to the bathroom. Yes, maybe we're a little more comfortable with physical issues of illness—because we've wiped a bottom or cleaned Jell-O off a chin. And maybe we're a little more comfortable considering our own mortality—because we've watched others deal with theirs and we see that—guess what?—dying isn't *completely* bad. Parts of it can be incredibly peaceful. Illuminating. Poignant. *Good,* in fact.

- **What we hospice volunteers *do* isn't so special.** The only difference between us and others is this—we simply *show up,* and do it.

NOTES

12

THE VISIT

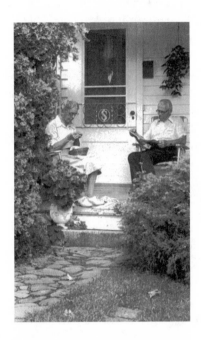

- **Call the family before your visit to confirm;** this builds trust and spares inconvenience. For instance, imagine that a patient is unexpectedly hospitalized. If the family knows the hospice worker phones before visits, there is one less responsibility on their shoulders.

- **Confirming phone calls also provide an additional opportunity to talk with patients and especially primary caregivers.** Not only will you be more prepared for the next visit, but in a private phone call the caregiver might be more willing to share those fears/feelings that are harder to discuss face-to-face, in the presence of the patient.

- **Bring something to do** on the visit (a good book, letters to write) for those times the family prefers to be left alone.

- **Things to bring in your hospice bag:** book, magazine, stationery and pen, surgical gloves, lotion for hand massages, handiwork, a snack, a journal, playing cards, tissues, emergency information.

- **Things to do on a hospice visit:** give the patient a manicure, apply makeup, write letters for the patient, read to the patient, massage, tidy the bathroom or kitchen, walk the dog, do grocery shopping or a pharmacy pickup, run errands, provide transportation to appointments, "chum" with the patient (cards, lunch, talk, country drives, looking at old photographs, sharing hobbies, etc.).

- **Most important thing to do on a hospice visit:** know when the client wants to be left alone.

- **Let the family control your visit.** When you arrive, ask: "What needs to be done today?"

- If the family doesn't seem to know what to do with you, **suggest something.** "Can I do a load of wash?" "Would a massage help?"

- Remember that **keeping out of the way** is sometimes the best thing you can do.

- A lot of hospice care consists of **being ingenious** in helping families solve their problems . . . from physical therapy issues like drinking from a glass to logistical issues like scheduling to emotional issues like reconciliations.

- **Be creative. Also be wary** of getting in over your head—be prepared to offer referrals.

- **Ask questions** of other team members when you have concerns.

- **Leave notes; share information** with other team members when you find something that works.

- **Each team member brings a unique perspective to the case, and each leaves a personal imprint with the family.**

NOTES

13

TAKING CARE
OF YOURSELF

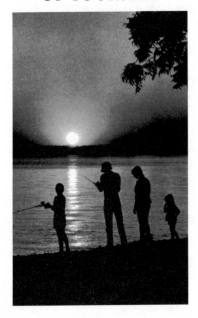

- **Pat yourself on the back for communicating at the very highest level possible.** (It requires tremendous skill and energy to ask the right questions, create trust, mediate, monitor airtime, read between the lines, reduce defensiveness . . . all simultaneously!)

- **Engage in stress-release activities:** exercise, journal writing, humor, hobbies, family rituals and traditions, eating well, rest, meditation, massage, outings with friends, spiritual nurturing, listening to relaxation tapes, music therapy, imagery exercises, bereavement support groups, storytelling, etc.

- **Hospice workers need respite, too.** Let your team members know when you need some time and distance.

- **Avoid judging or second-guessing your own reactions when patients die.** Crying profusely isn't necessarily overinvolvement; feelings of numbness don't necessarily mean that you are uncaring or burnt out.

- **Do not permit your own family and friends to put you on a pedestal because you are a hospice caregiver:** "You of *all* people should be strong enough to handle this . . . after all, you work with dying people!"

- **Don't worry about making mistakes.** I don't know of a caregiver in the world (even one with decades of experience) who can't think of a time when she wishes she'd said or done something differently.

- **Avoid feeling anxious even if it seems you are doing nothing.** In essence, you cannot change the family you are visiting, and you cannot change their circumstances. Your contribution is not what you *do*, but just that you are *there*.

- **Many times, it may seem as if you don't make a difference. But you do.**

NOTES

· 14 ·
EXERCISES FOR IMPROVING COMMUNICATION

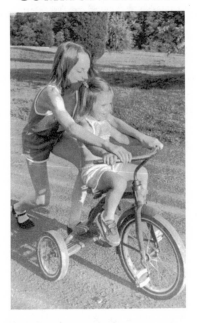

· **In this section you'll find several exercises designed to high-light important communication principles that are especially relevant to a hospice setting.** Use them in in-services. When appropriate, suggest them to the families you serve. Have fun with them, learn by them. Create your own communication exercises—above and beyond these starter ideas—ones that empha-size the most significant issues at your particular hospice program. Share your insights with your colleagues—at conferences, at in-services, and at team meetings.

"GENTLE" EXERCISES THAT FOSTER TRUST AND SELF-DISCLOSURE, AS WELL AS EMPHASIZE GROUP, TEAM, OR FAMILY COHESIVENESS

Choose an Object

Bring a box or bag of concealed objects—raid the desk, "junk drawer," garage, sewing box, kitchen, yard, etc., for small objects—about twice as many as the number of participants. Ask participants to sit in a circle. Have them come to the box, one-by-one, and choose an object with which they "identify." Give them a few moments to collect their thoughts, then have them share why they feel "connected" to that object. Ask them to focus on the values implied by their choices. Help them point out similarities and differences between members' choices, values, self-perceptions, etc.

Find a Gift

During a later, more intimate moment in your training, ask participants to go outside for half an hour and not talk to anyone at all. (Even if spoken to by others, they need to respond by merely smiling and nodding.) Ask them to think about themselves and the group and to search for a "gift" to bring back to their peers. The gift can be tangible (a beautiful stone, a leaf, a snack from the vending machines) or symbolic (a description of something they saw, an idea they had, a song). The important thing is that the gift represent something important for the giver and that it in some way expresses that person's feelings of togetherness as well as separateness from the group as a whole.

If the weather is inclement, the exercise can be performed inside, in hallways or lobbies, for example. But it works better if you can include nature.

The facilitator should also participate in this exercise. It is an excellent one for group bonding, and a nice way to "graduate" from volunteer training.

Structured Sharing

Exercises in self-disclosure are excellent methods for developing trust and learning about others' similarities and differences. There are lots of these exercises in self-help books and textbooks in interpersonal communication, but it is also very easy to write your own! Just type up a list of open-ended questions or incomplete sentences and custom-tailor them to your particular needs. A question or sentence needn't be complicated; in fact, more ambiguous items might work better. For example, "My mother . . ." puts fewer constraints on the participant than "My mother always treated me . . ." Blend "safe" items with more risky ones. For example, follow "A happy childhood memory . . ." with "I feel ashamed when . . ." See "Life Reveiw" Questions on page 89 for ideas.

You can make these exercises as short and sweet (five items, 15 to 20 minutes) or involved (scores of items, 2 to 3 hours) as your purposes dictate. The only rules are that (1) everything remains confidential; (2) participants do not have to answer any item that makes them uncomfortable; and (3) each person answers each item, in turn, before moving on to the next.

Participants typically feel great after this exercise. Many feel closer to someone else in the group than they thought possible, and they'll probably tell things they haven't spoken of in years.

How Do You Behave When . . .

Give participants 15 to 20 minutes to jot down their answers to the following (they will use these notes for discussion purposes only—no one will necessarily see their answers). As completely and specifically as you can, list the effect on your **language**, your **facial expression**, your **posture and gestures**, your **voice**, and the **way you dress** when you are:

	LANGUAGE	FACIAL EXPRESSION	POSTURE	GESTURES	VOICE	WAY YOU DRESS
NERVOUS						
CAREFREE						
ANGRY						
BORED						
DISAPPOINTED						
HAPPY						
AFFECTIONATE						
ENVIOUS						

List at least one effect on each of the characteristics (language, facial expression, etc.) for each of the eight emotional states above.

In a group discussion, share responses. Focus on expression of emotion and on similarities and differences between participants. Discuss the possible effects of culture on the responses. Do cultural differences affect the ways in which we express ourselves, especially certain emotions?

EXERCISES TO HELP PEOPLE EXPLORE THEIR
UPBRINGING AND FAMILY SYSTEMS

First Memories

Ask members to think about the very first memory they have—of a birthday celebration, their parents, their first friend, being judged by others, etc.

Choose a memory area (family, physical illness, loss, work, play, etc.) that pertains to the specific topics you'd like to cover in that training session.

Asking participants to recall their first memories of being a person of a particular gender, complexion, religion, ethnic group, or economic class makes a good diversity exercise.

Encourage members to share their memories in smaller groups of three to seven, then in a larger group of fifteen to twenty.

Ethical Wills

An exciting and meaningful in-service can be built around participants working on and discussing their personal ethical wills. This idea, originally adapted from the Jewish tradition of handing down legacies of values/beliefs/responsibilities, has been successfully used with our patient families. But how many team members have taken the time to explore this experience personally? An in-service like this will not only enhance your staff's understanding of their patients; it will also enable them to explore themselves and to locate similarities and differences between each other. Sharing the ethical wills as a group can also help build team cohesiveness.

Genograms

The tool we use in patient family assessment is wonderful for staff and volunteer in-services, too! An exciting session could be spent by explaining and creating genograms, thus giving participants the hands-on experience of charting their own genealogical relationships. Have them begin to build an understanding of their own family systems, emotions, cultural effects, loss issues, and isms. Sharing their self-insights in a discussion can also build trust in the group. If you are not familiar with this process, you can find a great step-by-step outline in *The Dance of Intimacy,* by Harriet Goldhor Lerner.

Warning: Some participants might have a more intense re-action to this exercise than you'd expect, especially if they suddenly recognize a pattern or an explanation for their own family dysfunction or loss issues. Be sure to leave plenty of time for processing and discussion.

EXERCISES TO HELP PEOPLE EXPRESS AND CLARIFY THEIR VALUES WHILE RECOGNIZING AND APPRECIATING THAT OTHERS HAVE DIFFERENT PERCEPTUAL FRAMEWORKS

Background Music

Choose any half hour when you want to convey some information in a lecture/discussion mode. But this time, play some lively music—quite audibly—in the background. If participants ask you about it, just say, "I'm hoping it will help. We'll talk about it later—let's just finish up this discussion first." Don't turn off the music, even if asked to, and don't explain yourself, either. After the half hour is up, ask what they thought about the music, if it was a distraction, if they felt frustrated because you refused to alter the environment (by turning off the music) when they asked you. The exercise is an excellent one for demonstrating how we become intolerant of others when they refuse to assimilate or do things the "proper" way.

I got this exercise idea from a Mexican-American man in my negotiations class who played loud salsa music during his presentation on Mexican-Anglo negotiations. I was distracted, frustrated, and tempted (as the instructor) to ask him to turn it down, if not off entirely. But something told me to hold my tongue. At the end of his presentation, he said, "Have you been noticing my music? Did it bother you? Well, I hope you managed to listen anyway, because if you ever try to negotiate in *my* country, with people like me, you'll be hearing this music everywhere. We play it all the time, and *loud.* And we would be very offended if you asked us to turn it off. So, get used to it, just like I have to adjust to too much quiet when I negotiate in the United States."

Directions: Give people a few moments to fill out this chart, then discuss it. The only rule is you *must* choose one of the three items.

I'd Rather

__ be wise	__ travel by plane	__ travel to Asia
__ be rich	__ travel by ship	__ travel to Europe
__ be attractive	__ travel by train	__ travel to Africa
__ be an only child	__ go skin-diving	__ be a surgeon
__ be the youngest child	__ go horseback riding	__ be an artist
__ be the oldest child	__ go snowmobiling	__ be a psychologist
__ lose my hearing	__ be a great singer	__ be very poor
__ lose my eyesight	__ be a great athlete	__ be very sickly
__ lose my legs	__ be a great actor	__ be very disfigured
__ be loyal	__ be selfish	__ spend money traveling
__ be generous	__ be a martyr	__ spend money on school
__ be honest	__ be apathetic	__ spend money on "toys"
__ live on a farm	__ lose economic freedom	__ be alone at work
__ live in the city	__ lose religious freedom	__ follow a leader at work
__ live in the suburbs	__ lose political freedom	__ lead the group at work
__ be by myself	__ live in the mountains	__ see relatives often
__ be with one friend	__ live in the desert	__ see relatives sometimes
__ be with acquaintances	__ live by the ocean	__ see relatives rarely
__ read the Bible	__ marry someone rich	
__ read Shakespeare	__ marry someone famous	
__ read history	__ marry someone healthy	

EXERCISES FOR EXPLORING TERRITORIAL SIMILARITIES, DIFFERENCES, ADJUSTMENTS

Proxemics

Clear a big space for movement, then ask half of the group to line up against one wall and the other half against the facing wall. The facilitator stands between the two lines, off to one side. Each member faces a specific partner across the room in the other line. Instruct partners to have a casual conversation from this distance (15 feet or more). After 60 seconds, ask participants each to step 2 feet forward (to 11 or more feet apart) and continue the conversation. After 60 seconds, again ask participants each to step 2 feet forward (to 7 or more feet apart) and continue the conversation. After 60 seconds, have them each step forward 1 foot (to 5 or more feet apart) and continue the conversation. Continue moving the groups closer every 60 seconds until they are literally inches apart. After the exercise, discuss comfort levels at various distances, nonverbal adjustments people made (e.g., intent eye contact when far apart, avoiding eye contact when at an intimate distance). Focus especially on cultural similarities and differences. Were some people more comfortable at a closer distance than others? Did some find the exercise funny, others anxiety-provoking?

Personal Space

Have participants take out a piece of paper and draw four concentric circles about ½ inch apart, the largest about 5 inches in diameter, the smallest about 2 inches in diameter. Label the circles 1 through 4. The circles represent Hall's distance zones: intimate distance (18 inches or less), personal distance (2 to 4 feet), social distance (4 to 12 feet) and public distance (12 feet or more).

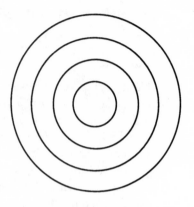

Then have participants indicate on the circles the degree of physical closeness they would feel comfortable with in the relationships/situations listed below. (For persons no longer living, recall what it was like to be physically near them and mark the distances you preferred when they were alive.) Discuss similarities and differences among participants' comfort levels. Are any cultural effects noticed?

Intimate zone:
18 inches or less—smallest circle
Personal zone:
2–4 feet—second smallest circle
Social zone:
4–12 feet—second largest circle
Public zone:
12 feet or more—largest circle

Place these initials on the circles where you would feel the distance is comfortable:

SO	= Strangers, opposite sex	B	= Brother
SS	= Strangers, same sex	FO	= Friend, opposite sex
O	= Older persons	FS	= Friend, same sex
K	= Kids, yours	T	= Teacher
KO	= Kids, others'	R	= Religious figure, clergy
CF	= Closest friend	LO	= Loved one/spouse
M	= Mother	TA	= Teenagers
F	= Father	L	= Friend laughing
S	= Sister	C	= Friend crying
		FA	= Friends arguing
		A	= Acquaintances arguing

MORE CONFRONTATIONAL EXERCISES—
ALSO ENLIGHTENING AND MEMORABLE

The Multiple Realities Exercise

This is a common and very effective exercise wherein participants are instructed, at the end of one training session, to go out into their lives and find an environment/event in which they are "different" from others, to "experience" that environment, then to write about it. At the next training session, the group can share their experiences. Some examples are attending a religious ceremony at a synagogue or temple if you are Christian, attending a cultural event sponsored by an ethnic group other than your own, going to a rock concert (must be post-eighties music!). Take care to instruct your participants to be respectful and wary of "bashing." This exercise could be dangerous, for instance, if someone goes to a gay bar only to gawk and giggle, besides possibly being unethical ("outing") or an invasion of privacy.

After everyone has taken a private field trip, regather for a group discussion. The group will have new insights about interpersonal comfort, trust, assimilation, group behavior, ritual, and the verbal/nonverbal ways we try to fit in.

Inclusion

Divide participants into groups of five to ten. Choose one person from each group, and instruct the other members to keep that person "outside" the group, using any verbal/nonverbal means necessary. This is an excellent (and sometimes scary) exercise that highlights assimilation, "shame of privilege," and the blame-the-victim phenomenon—all three will appear. It is important to keep participants in the groups well past the point of comfort (about 10 minutes) and it is also important to spend substantial time processing the experience (30 to 60 minutes). Otherwise people may leave feeling awful without gaining much insight.

The "Polar Words" Exercise

At your next in-service, spend 15 minutes with a diction-
ary! Pass out several and have teams look up and record the
meanings of opposites. Have one team record *health/illness,*
another *man/woman,* another *black/white,* another *life/death,*
another *husband/wife,* another *old/young.* Have the teams
read their definitions aloud. The entire group can recognize and discuss the various institutional isms in our language—ageism, sexism, racism, classism—and participants
will be able to appreciate the importance of "naming ourselves."

EXERCISES TO HIGHLIGHT THE DYNAMICS
OF LOSS AND GRIEF

The Loss Exercise

Give each participant sixteen blank index cards. (Or, if you have a large group, instruct each person to draw lines on a blank piece of paper to divide it into sixteen boxes.)

Ask each person to write something they love and value on each card (or box). It could be a person—one card for a spouse, other cards for each child and best friends. It could be a skill—driving, sewing, carpentry—or a possession—a wedding ring, a photograph, your mother's pearls. It could be an interest or hobby—singing, painting, gardening . . . anything at all the person feels is important in her life.

After each person has sixteen items, tell the participants to look at them and appreciate them for a few minutes. Then, tell them to take away four of the items—either by handing you the card or by drawing an X through four boxes. Ask them to consider—and share with each other—what it feels like to have these four things taken from their life.

Finally, walk around the room and randomly take four cards from each of the participants. (With a large group, have each person turn to his neighbor and randomly cross out four items on the other person's page.) Now ask them to consider again—and share with each other—what it feels like to be left with only eight of the original items. How do we compensate? What emotions do we experience? How was it different when they chose their losses, as opposed to when someone else randomly took away what they valued?

This is an incredibly powerful little exercise. Spend lots of time in discussion.

The Personal Grief Timeline

Draw a horizontal timeline like the one below on a piece of paper. (Provide yourself more space by turning the paper sideways first.) Starting with your birth and ending with the present:

- Place a dot—and note the date and your age—for each death you have experienced.
- Include the deaths of extended family, schoolmates, and pets.
- Also include the deaths of famous people, if they made an impact on you.
- For each death, note circumstances—accident, illness, age, suicide, war, etc.
- Also note the age of the person who died.

Birth . . . . *Today*

After you make your timeline, ask yourself some questions:

- *How many important relationships have you lost through death?*
- *Are these losses clustered during a particular time in your life?*
- *Do they appear in a pattern that proves enlightening?*
- *Do you have a lot of experience with a particular form of death—a specific illness, heart ailments, breast cancer, AIDS? Suicide? Miscarriage? War? Farm accidents?*
- *Have the people you've loved died old and happy? Young?*
- *How has all this experience contributed to who you are now?*
- *How do you feel today about death and dying, because of the deaths you've experienced (or have yet to experience)?*

"LIFE REVIEW" QUESTIONS:
GREAT TO USE WITH FAMILIES, HELPFUL THINGS TO ASK OUR CO-WORKERS — THE CONVERSATIONS THEY PROVOKE BUILD TRUST AND SELF-DISCLOSURE

Firsts

My first car . . .

My first job . . .

My first day of school . . .

My first success . . .

My first failure . . .

My first best friend . . .

My first kiss . . .

My first trip . . .

My first major illness . . .

My first memory . . .

My first time away from home . . .

Favorites

My very favorite things to do . . .

My very favorite place . . .

My favorite hobbies . . .

My favorite sports . . .

My favorite foods . . .

My favorite movies . . .

My favorite books . . .

My favorite TV shows . . .

My favorite actors/celebrities . . .

My favorite songs . . .

My favorite people . . .

My favorite colors . . .

My favorite time of day . . .

My favorite day of the week . . .

My favorite season . . .

My favorite year . . .

Family

My mother . . .

My father . . .

My siblings . . .

My grandparents . . .

Mother's family was . . .

Father's family was . . .

A favorite birthday celebration . . .

When I was little, we celebrated major holidays by . . .

My ancestry and ethnic heritage . . .

Our family's religious traditions were . . .

A favorite relative was . . .

A question I have about my family is . . .

The major values my parents tried to instill in me were . . .

When my spouse and I met . . .

I decided to get married because . . .

Our wedding was . . .

After my spouse and I had been married about ten years, I . . .

Some of the major tests of our marriage have been . . .

When I had my first (second, third, etc.) child, I . . .

When I was a young mother/father, I . . .

On holidays and birthdays we used to . . .

When the kids were little, I was really scared when . . .

Some funny or special stories about my children are . . .

Something about parenthood that has surprised me is . . .

Being a parent during the sixties (fifties, thirties, eighties, etc.) was . . .

When my kids were teenagers, I thought . . .

When I became a grandparent, I . . .

The way I feel today about my marriage is . . .

The major values I've tried to instill in my children are . . .

Growing Up

My hometown . . .

Growing up in (place) was . . .

Being born in the twenties (or thirties, fifties, seventies, etc.)
   meant that . . .

The house/s where I grew up was (were) . . .

Our neighborhood was . . .

When I was growing up, girls and women were . . .

When I was growing up, boys and men were . . .

As a child, some traditions that were always in place were . . .

On weekends we usually . . .

My earliest ambitions were . . .

Some childhood heroes were . . .

A secret place I had as a child was . . .

When I was little, I always dreamed that one day . . .

My parents usually disciplined me by . . .

I got in lots of trouble when . . .

My memories of my early school years are . . .

My favorite subjects in school were . . .

A favorite teacher was . . .

When I was little, something that really scared me was . . .

My favorite things to do as a kid were . . .

When I was a teenager, I used to . . .

The "fashions of the day" when I was young were . . .

When I was in college, I . . .

Some of my romantic interests have been . . .

Smells that remind me of my earlier years are . . .

Places I associate with my growing up are . . .

The special pets I remember are . . .

My best friends from elementary school were . . .

My best friends in high school were . . .

A childhood vacation I remember is . . .

A major embarrassing moment from childhood was . . .

A hard lesson I learned as a kid was . . .

A regret about my early years is . . .

When I was young, my family never knew I . . .

The people who helped me most when I was a young adult were . . .

When I was little, older people always said that I would . . .

When I was growing up, I always excelled at . . .

One of my fondest memories of childhood is . . .

Who Am I

Five adjectives that describe me are . . .

Other people would describe me as . . .

Friends who have known me for years say . . .

The issues and causes that get me stirred up are . . .

As I've grown older, I've changed in that . . .

If I could have a perfect week, it would be . . .

The way I prefer to dress is . . .

The way I look has changed over the years in that . . .

My voice . . .

In a group I usually . . .

Things I find funny are . . .

If I could have anything in the world, it would be . . .

If I could give any one thing in the world to any person in the world, I would give *(thing)* to *(person)* because . . .

Spiritually, I think of myself as . . .

The most important values I hold dear are . . .

If I could give one thing to the world, I'd give . . .

If I could leave one lesson for my children, it would be . . .

Peaks and Valleys

The best advice I ever received was . . .

My most embarrassing moment was . . .

I have always done better than others at . . .

The time I was most proud . . .

The most important experience of my life so far . . .

My major influences and mentors have been . . .

The worst boss I ever had was . . .

The biggest mistakes I've made have been . . .

I wish . . .

The projects that have given me the most pleasure are . . .

The thing I've had to work hardest at in my life is . . .

The one thing that makes me feel most alive is . . .

A major life regret is . . .

The hardest decision I've ever made . . .

One of the wisest things I've ever done is . . .

Some major hardships in my life have been . . .

The scariest time of my life was when . . .

The happiest times of my life have been . . .

The best thing I've ever done for someone else is . . .

The major blessings I've had are . . .

World View

Of all the places I've visited, I have the most vivid memories of . . .

I still want to travel to . . .

Some of my strongest memories regarding current events are . . .

In the 1920s . . .

During the Great Depression . . .

During World War II . . .

During the fifties . . .

During the sixties . . .

During the Vietnam War . . .

In the "me generation" decade . . .

My most memorable U.S. presidents have been . . .

Some major political events have been . . .

The most exciting political time of my life has been . . .

Some political causes that have always been important to me are . . .

Community and volunteer work I've done is . . .

The income-producing work I've done is . . .

I would define my career by saying . . .

Some famous people I've met . . .

Some "famous moments" I've had are . . .

To me, *art* means . . .

The natural disasters I remember are . . .

The world changes I've seen are . . .

My wishes for the world are . . .

THE IMPORTANCE OF PROCESSING

Communication training experiences can get intense. The skilled trainer will be sure to include specific structured mechanisms for participants to "process" what they have experienced. That way, people leave feeling like they learned something . . . not like they have just gotten beaten up. Here are some ideas:

Log Exercises

This is like a journal but is intentionally called a log to remove the "touchy-feely" psychological stigma. Also, participants are asked to write responses to structured questions rather than encouraged to use the tool for venting. For example, they may be told "Write about the nonverbal dynamics you just noticed in our discussion," rather than "Write about how you feel after that exercise." You can create specific log questions for participants to answer at home or use the exercise in class. You might ask a question and give participants 10 minutes to respond, in writing, before the discussion begins.

Free Writing

Ask participants a broad question, for example, "What did you learn, about yourself and about others, during that exercise?" Give them exactly three minutes to perform a freewriting exercise about it, and use the second hand on your watch to time them. Tell them, "It doesn't matter what you write; the only rule is that your pen has to be continually moving. Try to stay on the topic, but if you can't think of anything, just write 'I can't think of anything, I'm waiting to think of something,' until your creativity kicks in." This is a wonderful exercise for helping people "vent," especially after a particularly painful or scary discussion or exercise. Later, you can ask them to reflect on what they wrote and have a discussion.

Group Writing

This is a method a small group can use to process an experience together; each person writes one sentence, then hands the sheet to the next group member. The only rule is you can't write something that someone has already written. Keep passing the paper in the circle until no one has anything fresh or new to write. Then, read the entire document aloud.

The Ladder Technique

This exercise gives people a sense of accomplishment and closure at the end of a session, as well as ideas for their future journey. Tell people to pull out a piece of paper. You'll be asking them seven to nine open-ended statements or questions, giving them about 90 seconds to complete each one. Use the statements below, or create your own. Just be sure to have a positive and negative balance, and end on a positive, inspirational tone. You can collect these as evaluations, if you wish. A sample set of statements might include:

1. During this experience, I learned . . .
2. During this experience, I relearned . . .
3. After this experience, I still need to know . . .
4. The way I felt about myself during this experience was . . .
5. The way I felt about others during this experience was . . .
6. I regret that . . .
7. I'm happy about . . .
8. Other people need to know that . . .
9. I plan to continue with this learning by . . .

RESOURCES

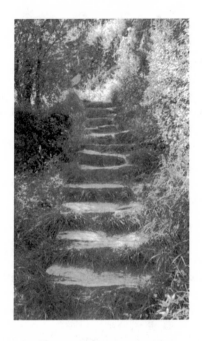

ORGANIZATIONS

- National Hospice Organization (NHO)
  1901 North Moore Street, Suite 901
  Arlington, VA 22209
  (703) 243-5900

- Hospice Nurses Association
  5512 Northumberland Street
  Pittsburgh, PA 15217
  (412) 687-3231

- Through reasonable membership and meaningful mailings, one has access to hospice periodicals, conference notices, video resources, books, support services, etc.

- Joining your state hospice organization is an excellent way to network and keep current on regional resources, workshops, and support.

ELECTRONIC SEARCH

Use the Internet and E-mail to obtain information and correspond with others. Use your community and college library databanks to obtain articles, books, and multimedia materials. Categories might be hospice, home-care, death, dying, bereavement, grief, palliative care, pain management, cancer, oncology, AIDS, terminal illness, family systems, conflict, neurolinguistics, personality, non-verbal communication, body language, etc.

BOOKS

There are far too many to list. Here is just a sample:

Achterberg, Jeanne, Barbara Dossey, and Leslie Kolkmeier. **Rituals of Healing: Using Imagery for Health and Wellness.** A wealth of practical insight and treatment for all sorts of illness pain—physical and otherwise.

Amenta, Madalon, and Nancy Bohnet. **Nursing Care of the Terminally Ill.** The award-winning classic, thorough, definitive, and guaranteed to instill confidence in any practitioner (perhaps out of print/contact Hospice Nurse Associations for information).

Beissler, Arnold R. **A Graceful Passage.** Essays and personal reflections on living and the right to die; how and when one chooses.

Benson, Herbert, and Miriam Klipper. **The Relaxation Response.** Information and techniques of meditation, helpful for stress reduction in patient families as well as for hospice workers.

Beresford, Larry. **The Hospice Handbook.** What hospice is, what it isn't, asking the right questions, finding hospice care; an early classic in the field of hospice.

Berg, Elizabeth. **Family Traditions: Celebrations for Holidays and Everyday.** A nonfiction work, practical and beautifully presented; great ideas for families who wish to enhance life.

Berg, Elizabeth. **Talk Before Sleep.** A beautiful novel about a hospice situation and the handful of friends who experience it together.

Borger, Irene, ed., **From a Burning House.** A sizable collection of stories, prose, and poetry written by people who have firsthand experience with HIV and AIDS. Some pieces are funny, some are heart-wrenching, and nearly all will help the reader celebrate the human spirit.

Buscaglia, Leo. **The Fall of Freddy the Leaf: A Story of Life for All Ages.** A tale of the life of a leaf with full-color photos; good way to orient kids to life's cycles.

Callanan, Maggie, and Patricia Kelley. **Final Gifts.** A beautifully written book which helps us appreciate the symbolic communication and metaphors used by patients with 'Nearing Death Awareness'; tuning into these metaphors can enhance patient-family relationships.

Carroll, David. **Living with Dying: A Loving Guide for Family and Close Friends.** Helpful, solid info, reader-friendly, written in a question-answer format.

Carter, Rosalynn, with Susan K. Golant. **Helping Yourself Help Others.** A helpful definition of caregiving . . . excellent resource lists—pages of organizations and a bibliography, by condition.

Childs-Gowell, Elaine. **Good Grief Rituals: Tools for Healing.** Short, sweet, and pragmatic; ideas to immediately implement, for finding hope, healing, and meaning.

Duda, Deborah. **Coming Home: A Guide to Dying at Home with Dignity.** A highly practical, comforting, and inspiring guidebook for home caregivers—a great book for patients and families.

Feinstein, David, and Peg Elliott Mayo. **Rituals for Living and Dying.** How we can turn loss and the fear of death into an affirmation of life; a book of tools, insights, and stories.

Fisher, Mary. **I'll Not Go Quietly.** A collection of talks by the famous AIDS patient/activist.

Fisher, Mary. **My Name Is Mary.** The author/activist's most recent, her memoirs.

Fisher, Mary. **Sleep with the Angels.** More talks by the AIDS patient/activist.

Ford, Michael Thomas, editor. **The Voices of AIDS: Twelve Unforgettable People Talk About How AIDS Has Changed Their Lives.**

Fry, Virginia Lynn. **Part of Me Died, Too: Stories of Creative Survival Among Bereaved Children and Teenagers.** Helpful and beautifully written narratives of children experiencing grief.

Galanti, Geri-Ann. **Caring for Patients from Different Cultures.** An enlightening anecdotal account of culture and sensitivity in a medical setting.

Gray, John. **Men Are From Mars, Women Are From Venus.** The best-seller about improving interpersonal communication, particularly between the sexes.

Greif, Judith, and Beth Ann Golden. **AIDS Care at Home: A Guide for Caregivers, Loved Ones, and People with AIDS.** An excellent handbook, full of information especially about physical care.

Grollman, Earl A. A prolific and charismatic rabbi and psychologist who specializes in grief. Some of his many titles include: **Living When a Loved One Has Died, Talking About Death: A Dialogue Between Parent and Child,** and **Straight Talk About Death for Teenagers: How to Cope with Losing Someone You Love.**

Gunther, John, **Death Be Not Proud: A Memoir.** A father's poignant story of his teenaged son's courageous battle with a brain tumor. Because Johnny's death occurred in 1947, this book additionally provides a historical view of how a child's illness may have been handled 50 years ago versus today.

Imber-Black, Evan, and Janine Roberts. **Rituals for Our Times: Celebrating, Healing, and Changing Our Lives and Our Relationships.** An in-depth overview of rituals with exercises for creating them, examining the self, and finding new meaning.

Irish, Donald, with Kathleen Lundquist and Vivian Nelson. **Ethnic Variations in Dying, Death, and Grief.** One of the first comprehensive volumes on culture and dying.

Karnes, Barbara. **Gone from My Sight: The Dying Experience.** A pithy pamphlet that outlines the physical and mental changes that occur as death approaches from 1 to 3 months, 1 to 2 weeks, days, hours, and minutes. Send $2.00 to Barbara Karnes, P.O. Box 335, Stilwell, KS 66085.

Karnes, Barbara. **A Time to Live: Living with a Life-threatening Illness.** A short and comforting little pamphlet for newly diagnosed people. Send $2.00 to Barbara Karnes, P.O. Box 335, Stilwell, KS 66085.

Keirsey, David, and Marilyn Bates. **Please Understand Me.** Info on Myers-Briggs.

Kramer, Kay, and Herbert Kramer. **Conversations at Midnight: Coming to Terms with Dying and Death.** A married couples' dialogues about living with illness; the wife is a social worker specializing in grief work, the husband a communications consultant who has incurable cancer.

Kübler-Ross, Elisabeth. Perhaps the most highly renowned—and controversial—expert on the subject of death and dying, Kübler-Ross is also a prolific writer on the subject, beginning in the sixties with her classic **On Death and Dying** and more recently writing **AIDS: The Ultimate Challenge.** Her numerous books are unique, from interviews and poignant photojournalism to highly technical, clinical descriptions. Her voice is penetrating and far-reaching.

Larson, Dale G. **The Helper's Journey.** Excellent information on caregiver stress and self-care.

Lerner, Harriet Goldhor. **The Dance of Intimacy, the Dance of Anger, the Dance of Deception.** A trio of great insights, family therapies, and genogram information.

Moore, Thomas. **Care of the Soul.** A warm and comforting book which encourages us to find depth and sacredness in everyday life. And more recently by Moore, **Soul Mates—Honoring the Mysteries of Love and Relationship.**

Morse, Melvin, with Paul Perry. **Closer to the Light.** A ground-breaking best-seller which put the notion of the Near Death Experience (NDE) into our vernacular and made us all consider just how wonderful dying might feel.

Morse, Melvin, with Paul Perry. **Transformed by the Light.** Continued research on people who have had NDEs shows them to be profoundly changed for the better, for the rest of their lives—with greater peace, zest for living, less fear of death, etc.

Moyers, Bill. **Healing and the Mind.** In book form, the famed PBS series appears as interviews and articles by experts the world over, who explore the mind-body connection and its healing powers.

Nuland, Sherwin B. **How We Die: Reflections on Life's Final Chapter.** A physician's descriptions of body-system shutdowns, from deaths of various causes.

Osis, Karl, and Erlendur Haraldsson. **At the Hour of Death.** A clinical overview of the death experience; deathbed visions, apparitions, depression, pain, and back from death experiences. Good source citation.

Patton, Marvyl Loree. **Guide-lines and God-lines for Facing Cancer.** A spiritual and practical book about living with serious illness; inspiring without preaching.

Quindlen, Anna. **One True Thing.** A gripping novel about a woman caring for her dying mother; she's later accused of 'euthanizing' her. . . . Excellent insights into family dynamics and ethics of incurable illness.

Rando, Therese. **How to Go on Living When Someone You Love Dies.** A classic text on loss and surviving it, from one of the nation's most respected experts.

Rando, Therese. **Treatment of Complicated Mourning.** A more recent contribution, warmly written yet highly clinical and helpful.

Rosen, Eliot J. **Families Facing Death: Family Dynamics of Terminal Illness.**

Rudd, Andrea, and Darien Taylor, editors. **Positive Women— Voices of Women Living with AIDS.** A collection of writing, poetry, and interviews with thirty-seven women with AIDS, who hail from all over the world.

Sachs, Judith. **When Someone You Love Has AIDS: A Dell Caregivers Guide.** A handy paperback, full of clinical information, other resources, and more.

Sankar, Andrea. **Dying at Home: A Family Guide for Caregiving.** Well written, practical, lots of info on physical care—helpful to a medical novice caregiver.

Sarton, May. **A Reckoning.** A poignant novel which traces the final year of Laura Spellman, who is diagnosed with inoperable lung cancer. She takes over the helm of her illness and comes to terms with her life and her relationships.

Stoddard, Sandol. **The Hospice Movement: A Better Way of Caring for the Dying.** An early and important classic about hospice care and its development.

Stone, Richard. **Stories: The Family Legacy, A Guide for Recollection and Sharing.** A brief and beautifully produced pamphlet on methods for drawing out the stories in those we love; contact Story Work Institute at (407) 767-0067.

Tannen, Deborah. **You Just Don't Understand** and **That's Not What I Meant.** A sociolinguist looks at language use, with major emphasis on gender differences; a forerunner to John Gray.

Tolstoy, Leo, **The Death of Ivan Ilyich.** A short little novel by the Russian master, considered by many to be one of the finest fictional accounts of illness and dying. Tolstoy tells the story of a privileged man who has never given much thought to his own existence until he is forced to come face-to-face with his own mortality.

von Oech, Roger. **A Kick in the Seat of the Pants** and **A Whack on the Side of the Head.** Two highly practical, helpful, and fun books on creativity and idea generation. Also available as a **"Whack Pack"**—a handy deck of Tarot-sized cards, each with a different creativity tip, idea, or sparkler. Use the cards at family and team meetings.

White, E. B. **Charlotte's Web.** This is the classic children's novel about Wilbur the pig and his best friend, Charlotte the spider, who teaches Wilbur about life, death, and that love is eternal. A wonderful read-aloud book for family members of all ages, and a good way to introduce children to that which is sacred in life's passages.

Worden, William. **Grief Counseling and Grief Therapy.** A classic examination of the grief process, quite clinical yet warmly written, accessible to the layperson.

ABOUT THE AUTHOR

M. Catherine Ray is a hospice educator, author, and volunteer. She provides workshops all over the nation and is a frequent presenter at conferences hosted by the National Hospice Organization. Catherine holds a B.A. magna cum laude in interpersonal communications, and a master's degree in speech communication. Since 1977 she has taught college-level courses in interpersonal communications, negotiation, and public speaking. In 1991 she was honored by students with the Excellence in Teaching award at Metropolitan State University, Saint Paul, Minnesota.

In 1984 Catherine began to specialize in hospice communication, traveling throughout the region to provide hospice workers with training in patient-family communication. She began writing in the early 90's; her articles and book reviews have appeared in *Hospice Magazine* and the *American Journal of Nursing*. After becoming a hospice volunteer herself, Catherine was ready to write *I'm Here to Help: A Hospice Worker's Guide to Communicating with Dying People and Their Loved Ones*.

After completing *I'm Here to Help*, Catherine's immediate dream was to write an expanded version—for patients and loved ones rather than for those who help the family professionally. *I'm With You Now* was begun in 1993. A year later, Catherine's husband was diagnosed with a rare lymphoma. She hopes her family's experience with incurable illness is enlightening rather than self-indulgent.

Catherine lives with her husband and daughter near Minneapolis. The family enjoys travel, boating, biking, and music.

If you feel

I'm Here to Help

is an important book for the
hospice profession,
then you'll feel
M. Catherine Ray's
next book

I'm With You Now

A GUIDE THROUGH INCURABLE ILLNESS
FOR PATIENTS, FAMILIES, AND FRIENDS

is equally important for patients,
families, and friends of those suffering
from incurable illness.

Eminently practical, *I'm With You Now* explains to
those closest to the patient how best to communicate,
be helpful and supportive, and deal with the frustrations
and sadness that inevitably accompany any
hospice environment.

A Bantam trade paperback available now